THE GREEK YOGURT DIET

Lose Belly Fat and Get Slim Now

James Guetzkow, M.D.
Jason Guetzkow

Many of the designations used by manufacturers and sellers to distinguish their products are claimed as trademarks. Where those designations appear in this book and the authors were aware of the trademark claim, the designations have been printed in initial capital letters.

First paperback edition 2013

ISBN: 1-4839-9795-2
ISBN-13: 978-1-4839-9795-7

Note: This book is intended only as an informative guide for those wishing to know more about health issues. In no way is this book intended to replace, countermand or conflict with the advice given to you by your own physician. The ultimate decision concerning care should be made between you and your doctor. We strongly urge you to follow the advice of your physician. Information in this book is general and is offered with no guarantees on the part of the authors. The authors disclaim all liability in connection with the use of this book.

SECTION 1

THE GREEK YOGURT DIET

CHAPTER 1

WHAT'S THE STORY WITH GREEK YOGURT?

Remember the famous line delivered by Gordon Gekko in the 1987 movie *Wall Street?* "Greed works." Well, it turns out that there is excellent news for our waistlines that can be summed up by an equally succinct statement. *Yogurt works.* While we might want to get someone other than Gordon Gekko to deliver that line for us, perhaps someone like a friendly dairy farmer, the good news needs to be heard by everyone.

It might surprise you to learn that yogurt has humble origins. It was probably invented accidentally by ancient peoples living in the Middle East. What most likely happened is that some milk unintentionally came in contact with a group of live cultures called *L. bulgaricus.* The live cultures may have been living on the surface of some random plant, and then possibly transferred by the hands of the person responsible for milking animals so that it was able to make contact with some milk.

When *L. bulgaricus* acts on milk, a biological process results in the creation of yogurt. It is theorized that once those ancient peoples attempted over the course of one or more days to eat what had been created, they almost immediately recognized that their new discovery would allow them to better preserve milk. In the days that long predated refrigeration, the discovery of yogurt represented a giant leap forward. Yogurt does not spoil as fast as milk under warm conditions. Therefore, it is believed that when people first produced yogurt intentionally, they employed the cultured milk product for utilitarian rather than culinary purposes.

One rather colorful legend claims that yogurt first came about in the 12th century when a group of villagers in Turkey wanted to send an angry message back to Genghis Khan, the Mogul emperor. According to the story, a messenger on horseback was sent on his way back to Khan with a gourd filled with milk rather than the water that it was supposed to carry. Instead of spoiling the gourd's cargo as the villagers had intended, the desert heat combined with the gallop of the steed and activated the milk. As a result, yogurt was created. The story is almost certainly a work of fiction, though an entertaining one.

You might ask, "Well, if yogurt goes back to ancient times in the Middle East, then what's the story with Greek yogurt?" Well, yogurt made its way into Greece thousands of years ago, and it has played a role in Greek culture ever since. In accordance with ancient customs, Greek newlyweds typically eat yogurt with honey and walnuts in order to ensure that they receive the celestial gifts of prosperity and energy before going on their honeymoons. However, this practice may have more

2

to do with the fact that people in Greece have long viewed yogurt as an aphrodisiac than anything else. Yogurt has served as a staple of Greek cuisine for a very long time, and it is popular there today. In just the past few years, frozen yogurt shops have started to open in Greece, putting a modern twist on an ancient delicacy.

In Greece, yogurt has always been made from the milk of a sheep or a goat while, in America, Greek yogurt is made from cow's milk. The Greek style of making yogurt varies from the methods used previously in the Middle East in one critical way. The process for making Greek yogurt is identical to those used previously to make yogurt, except that the finished product undergoes one final step. At the very end, the watery content of the yogurt is strained out in order to give Greek yogurt its thick texture.

Traditionally, Greek yogurt came only in its full fat form, but it has been modernized to give us low-fat and non-fat varieties. Greek yogurt has been touted as having a richer and creamier texture that makes it even more enjoyable to eat than regular yogurt. More important than Greek yogurt's taste and feel, however, is the superiority of its nutrient profile.

Greek yogurt has a number of key nutritional advantages over regular (non-Greek) yogurt due to its preparation method. Greek yogurt has approximately twice the protein of regular yogurt. Greek yogurt also has more calcium. Additionally, it contains less lactose than regular yogurt. Lactose is the type of naturally occurring sugar found in milk. Finally, Greek yogurt has fewer carbohydrates than regular yogurt.

This book represents our desire to accomplish four goals, each in its own section. Section 1 of this book tells the story of how yogurt has been scientifically proven to help you achieve your weight-loss goals. Section 2 helps you to change your lifestyle so that being healthy will become second nature to you. Section 3 of this book ensures that you start out with a basic diet that promotes good health and makes weight loss easier to achieve. Section 4 provides you with direct steps that will lead you to reduce your caloric intake and integrate Greek yogurt into your diet in the way that works best for you.

CHAPTER 2

YOGURT WORKS

The research indicates that yogurt ignites the body's ability to burn fat, accelerates weight loss, maintains both bone density and lean muscle mass and trims the stubborn fat around the middle of our bodies, according to a study published in the *International Journal of Obesity*.

The study looked at obese adults eating three servings of fat-free yogurt a day as part of a reduced-calorie diet. To give this some perspective, a single serving of yogurt is one cup, and so those participating in the test group ate three cups of yogurt per day. Those obese adults dropped 22% more weight and **61% more body fat** than those who reduced caloric intake but failed to eat yogurt. They also dropped **81% more fat in the stomach area** than non-yogurt eaters.

"Not only did yogurt help the study participants lose more weight—the average weight loss was 14 pounds—they were about twice as effective at maintaining lean muscle mass," stated researcher Michael Zemel, PhD, professor of nutrition at the University of Tennessee, in a news release. "This is a critical issue when dieting—you want to lose fat, not muscle. Muscle helps burn calories, but it is often compromised during weight loss."

It is important to emphasize that while all of the subjects lost weight due to a reduction of their total caloric intake, the study showed that both weight and fat loss were significantly greater in the yogurt group. For example, those on the non-yogurt diet lost an average of 11 pounds while those on the yogurt diet lost an average of more than 14 pounds.

From a health standpoint, one of the biggest findings of the study is that subjects on the yogurt diet lost 81% more fat in the stomach area. This is important because "visceral fat" (within the abdomen) is the most dangerous type of fat. A portion of the excess fat in the middle of our bodies, that gives the body an "apple shape," has been tied to an increased risk of heart disease, diabetes, stroke and even some forms of cancer. Visceral fat constantly returns fatty acids into bloodstream circulation, while "pear-shaped" obesity below the waistline stores and isolates fat away from the bloodstream. Keep visceral fat in mind when we later learn that the stress hormone called *cortisol* tends to dangerously increase fat stores in the middle of our bodies.

If you simply looked at the facts about yogurt, you might conclude that yogurt looks a lot like exercise by the spoonful. Yogurt causes us to lose fat while maintaining lean body mass just like exercise. Can you imagine what people would pay for a pill they could take that would give them the benefits of exercise without having to break a sweat? Yogurt is downright cheap compared to what people would pay for an exercise pill, and you can buy yogurt just about anywhere and do so without a prescription.

We are not recommending the Greek Yogurt Diet in place of exercise. Exercise serves as a vital and necessary component of the Greek Yogurt Diet program. Moreover, exercise will help you to maintain, for the rest of your life, the weight loss that you achieve by following the Greek Yogurt Diet. We are merely comparing the Greek Yogurt Diet to exercise in order to point out how powerful the diet can be and what a pivotal factor it can play in both improving and maintaining your health.

CHAPTER 3

HOW YOGURT WORKS

While yogurt has been proven to help you lose weight, there are competing theories that try to explain exactly how yogurt works. While it is possible that only one of the theories is correct, it is more likely that multiple mechanisms are working together to make yogurt effective. It will take future studies to discover the exact mechanisms at play that result in yogurt's effectiveness. In the meantime, eat your yogurt. It works.

CALCIUM

As we have discussed, a study was published in the *International Journal of Obesity* that evaluated yogurt as a weight-loss treatment (see Chapter 1 above). The study's author, Michael Zemel, suggested that it was the calcium content of yogurt that maintains bone density and muscle mass while increasing fat loss. It is worth noting that Greek yogurt may boast of even more calcium than the regular yogurt that was used in the study.

While the calcium content of yogurt may have played a role in preserving bone density, there are no studies showing that consuming calcium above the recommended daily allowance leads to weight loss. There are only studies showing that a diet that is deficient in calcium may lead to obesity, and that curing a deficiency in calcium may lead to weight loss.

There is also no study that compares the intake of calcium from an isolated supplement (such as in a pill) with an equal quantity of calcium taken in the form of yogurt as a treatment for calcium deficiency. We believe that such a study would show that the group of subjects getting their calcium from yogurt would lose weight, especially from the middle of their bodies, while maintaining their bone density and muscle mass. Meanwhile, the group of subjects taking a calcium supplement would only experience the maintenance of bone density, comparatively modest weight loss with no increased loss of belly fat and a greater loss of muscle mass. To sum it up, the subjects eating yogurt would be enjoying those benefits of yogurt that go far beyond the benefits to be had due to yogurt's calcium content.

> # IMPORTANT HEALTH ALERT
>
> Not only is there no evidence showing that excessive calcium intake can result in weight loss, there is new and mounting evidence showing that too much dietary calcium can lead to heart problems. It is important that you discuss the amount of calcium that you are taking with your doctor. It may turn out that you will get all of your calcium needs met simply by eating yogurt, and do not need to take supplements. If you are concerned about osteoporosis, please also discuss osteoporosis prevention and treatment with your physician before doing something potentially harmful such as excessively consuming calcium through supplements.

PROBIOTICS ARE ONE HOT TOPIC

Probiotics are the live microorganisms that are thought to be helpful to people, and they have become an exceptionally hot topic in popular health right now. In fact, more than one line of yogurt products has been rolled out in order to cash in on all of the hype surrounding probiotics. And if you open up the pages of a health magazine, you are likely to find a discussion on the myriad health benefits of the probiotics found in yogurt and other food sources.

Research has demonstrated that one strain of probiotics has been found to lower bad cholesterol by nearly 12% and reduce total and saturated cholesterol esters that contribute to the hardening of arteries. Probiotics may be effective in the treatment of a wide variety of ailments of the digestive system. Surprisingly, probiotics have even been found to prevent respiratory illness, and may even cut the recovery time for people suffering from the common cold. One recent study even indicates that some probiotics may curb certain features of depression and anxiety.

While there is a lot of research in support of the potential health benefits of having the right balance of bacteria and other microbes in the gut, the benefits of probiotics ingested from food may have been slightly overstated. The reason is, in part, that most of the probiotics found in foods do not survive the harsh digestive acids of the stomach. Also, some of the probiotics found in food do not continue to multiply in the colon. This means that as soon as you stop taking the probiotics they disappear from your body. Finally, there may not be a sufficient quantity of probiotics present in food sources to actually have an effect in the gut.

It should be noted that a certain percentage of the probiotics found in yogurt may make it past the stomach and thrive in the intestines (gut). The exact amount that make it will vary depending upon the strain of probiotics, the conditions in your stomach at the time that the probiotics pass through it and how much of the bacteria is actually present in the yogurt or other food that you are eating. However, due to the possible limitations of probiotics ingested in this manner, you should not rely on yogurt and other foods as your only source. You should also seek out probiotics that have been freeze-dried because they have a much better chance of reaching the gut and thriving there.

You should be able to obtain freeze-dried probiotics in the form of capsules or tablets from your local pharmacy, and they should be available as an over-the-counter supplement. While the health benefits of the probiotics available over-the-counter are still being proven as of this writing, we expect that the effectiveness of such products will only improve over time as further research is being conducted that will guide which probiotics get included in future formulations.

We recommend taking a freeze-dried probiotic that has several types of beneficial bacteria. Importantly, the label should state that the presence of the bacteria has been scientifically confirmed. Speak to your pharmacist if you have any trouble finding freeze-dried probiotics. It may be a good idea to take some when you start the diet to ensure that you have enough of the beneficial bacteria and other microbes in your gut at the outset. Then, the microbes living in your gut may be conditioned by the introduction of the complex sugars present in yogurt (see the discussion on good sugars below).

Research may also someday show that it is possible to assist weight loss by altering the composition of microbes found in the digestive system. Some researchers speculate that, in the future, probiotics will be tailor-made for each individual's specific needs. If you want to lose weight, a combination of probiotics and possibly antibiotics will be assembled for you in just the right sequence and combination in order to condition your gut microbes to help you best achieve weight loss. In the meantime, you may want to both eat yogurt and supplement with freeze-dried probiotics in light of the fact that science has shown that probiotics can have beneficial effects on your health.

GOOD SUGARS

In addition to promoting probiotics directly into the gut, there is another way to have an impact on the balance of bacteria and other microbes that exist in the digestive system. Certain types of complex sugars may make it past the stomach and help the right kinds of helpful bacteria and other microbes already present in the gut to thrive. These complex sugars can be described as prebiotics.

HELPFUL HINT

It is important to emphasize that we are not saying that simple sugars can be good for you. We are only talking about the potential health benefits of *complex* sugars. In order to make sure that you are avoiding simple sugars, check the nutrition facts on food labels. The grams of sugar contained in a single serving of each product can be found under the heading "Total Carbohydrate." The amount of sugar shown refers to both naturally occurring sugars and added sugars. Choose products that have as little sugar as possible.

While the words prebiotics and probiotics look alike and are related terms, they describe two very different things. Probiotics are the bacteria and other microbes that are thought to promote health. Prebiotics are food ingredients that cannot be absorbed through our intestines and, instead, are digested by certain classes of gut bacteria that work together.

Yogurt may contain the types of prebiotics that promote the growth and activity of bacteria and other microbes found in the digestive system in ways that are thought to be good for our health. The starting point for yogurt is milk. Mammals have developed the adaptation to produce a milk that perfectly meets the health needs of their offspring, including their offspring's need for a good balance of bacteria and other microbes in the gut. Through a biological process, milk containing prebiotics is then made into a yogurt that retains the prebiotic content of the milk. We may, therefore, obtain prebiotics by eating yogurt.

One type of prebiotic that may be found in yogurt comes in the form of the complex sugars called fructooligosaccharides (pronounced frook-toe-ah-lee-go-SACK-uh-rides) or FOS for short. FOS are certain types of fibers that are not digested in the stomach. Once in the gut, they appear to have the ability to both reduce harmful organisms on the one hand, and boost the growth of health-promoting bacteria and other microbes on the other. But the presence of FOS in yogurt is not the only factor behind the amazing weight-loss benefits seen with yogurt. The most significant factor has to do with protein.

THE PROTEIN FACTOR

Before we examine the exact types of proteins found in yogurt, let us consider the role that protein, in general, can play in weight loss. The *American Journal of Clinical Nutrition* published a study in which the participants reported greater satisfaction, suffered less from hunger, and had more weight

15

loss when the fat in their diet was reduced to 20% of their total caloric intake, protein was stepped up to 30% and carbohydrates accounted for 50% of their caloric intake. While they were allowed to determine their own calorie intake, those in the test group consumed 441 less calories per day on the high-protein diet. This means that they were allowed to eat as much as they wanted but chose to eat significantly less due to their increased protein consumption.

The weight loss experienced by the test group shows us that adequate protein intake can make a huge difference in appetite control. All other things being equal, by eating non-fat, Greek yogurt, you will be stepping up your protein intake significantly, even beyond the amount of protein that you would get from regular (non-Greek) yogurt. At the same time, by eating non-fat Greek yogurt, you will also be reducing your overall fat intake and consumption of carbohydrates.

It is important to keep in mind that fat intake is critically important. You do not want to eliminate fat in all forms from your diet. Your goal is simply to remove bad fat from your diet and to replace it with health-promoting fats, primarily Omega-3 fatty acids and monounsaturated fat. Later in this book, we will show you ways to accomplish these tasks that are both nutritious and delicious. But first, let us take a look at the primary mechanism that makes yogurt so effective for weight loss.

THE POWER OF WHEY

It appears that the chief reason for the effectiveness of the cultured dairy product known as yogurt is its extremely high whey protein content. Whey protein is a type of protein found in milk and dairy products. The exact amount of whey protein varies from dairy product to dairy product. For instance, most cheeses have low amounts of whey protein, but ricotta cheese has somewhat greater amounts of whey protein, although it has less than yogurt. Also, while yogurt is generally high in whey protein, different manufacturing processes result in levels of whey protein that vary from brand to brand. Unfortunately, certain brands of Greek yogurt offer less whey protein than other. This makes it important to do your homework before choosing your preferred brand or brands of Greek yogurt. Let us now take a close look at the research into the effects of whey protein.

A 2006 study showed that whey protein can be effective for weight loss even at a normal caloric intake, while soy protein causes the body to maintain its current body weight at the same number of calories. The study, conducted at the U.S. Department of Agriculture's Human Nutrition Research Center, took 90 overweight, middle-aged adults and put them into one of three groups. The first group added whey protein drinks to their otherwise normal diets, the second group added soy protein drinks and the last group drank drinks solely containing carbohydrates. This experiment showed that whey protein might be superior for weight-loss purposes when compared to soy protein and perhaps to other kinds of protein.

After six months, people drinking the carbohydrate shakes had gained about 2 pounds, which appeared to consist mainly of an increase in fat rather than an increase in lean body mass. People drinking the soy shakes neither gained nor lost weight.

People drinking the whey protein, in contrast, had successfully lost a little bit of weight and body fat, about 2 pounds. But even more significantly, those consuming the whey protein **lost about an inch around the middle of their bodies.**

The results of this line of research tell us that, for the purpose of losing weight, whey protein is the protein of choice. And, as we are about to learn, one type of whey protein in particular— and its ability to reduce cortisol levels in your body—is the key.

The success of whey protein begs the question: Why is whey protein more effective for weight loss than all other kinds of protein? It turns out that the whey protein derived from milk that may be present in yogurt is high in alpha-lactalbumin (pronounced AL-fa-lack-tall-BOOM-in). Alpha-lactalbumin is a type of whey protein that acts directly on cortisol levels. In a study published in the *American Journal of Clinical Nutrition*, researchers from the TNO Nutrition and Food Research Institute in the Netherlands examined the impact of alpha-lactalbumin on cortisol levels under stress by looking at vulnerable subjects. Researchers found that people consuming a diet rich in alpha-lactalbumin enjoyed reductions in cortisol levels after undergoing a short period of stress in contrast to people consuming a diet high in casein protein (another protein found in milk) who did not enjoy reductions in cortisol levels.

Now that we know that whey protein acts on cortisol, let us take a quick look at what cortisol is and how it affects our health. In order to avoid confusion, we should first note that cortisol is sometimes referred to as cortisone or hydrocortisone. Cortisol is a naturally occurring hormone, and it is essential for normal functioning. Among its many roles, cortisol can act as a powerful anti-inflammatory agent. Cortisol is released from the adrenal glands when the body is beset with physical or psychological stress in order to assist with controlling the immune system and to help control the body's sleep cycles. Cortisol plays a role in the so-called Dawn Effect that helps us to awaken when we rise to meet a challenging day. As a "first responder" to stress, cortisol is also involved in the body's fight-or-flight response.

Think of the body as a machine that has no way to differentiate between sources of stress. When your heart rate accelerates from physical activity, your body has no idea if there is a recreational cause for the increase (like going for a bike ride) or if there is a hazardous event to blame (like running because you are being chased). As far as the body is concerned, any level of exercise is interpreted as a stressful event and without proper conditioning through regular exercise your body will release cortisol in response. This is one reason why exercise is so critical for our health.

When called into action, the stress hormone called cortisol makes sources of energy (sugar in the form of glucose) ready for use by first causing the liver to manufacture more sugar and then causing sugar to be stored as glycogen. Next, cortisol blocks insulin from reducing glucose levels (glucose is the type of sugar found in the bloodstream). When insulin cannot act on glucose, the glucose is not stored in muscles and so it builds up in the bloodstream. Cortisol also causes proteins and fats to be broken down and used for energy. The problem with all of this is that unless you are exercising, much of this glucose, together with the stripped-down protein and broken-down fat that are left over from this process, will eventually get turned into fat and stored inside fat cells.

While cortisol in normal levels is necessary for healthy functioning, excessive cortisol levels can have a disastrous effect on our bodies. Due to its ability to halt protein synthesis and turn calories into fat, too much of this hormone can make us gain weight. Simply put, the more cortisol in our bodies, the more overweight we tend to be. To get a better handle on how this hormone acts on our bodies, let us look at Cushing's syndrome. Cushing's is also known as hypercorticism (which essentially translates as "overly high levels of cortisol").

Cushing's syndrome may be described as the sum of symptoms associated with long-term exposure to high levels of cortisol. Or, to put it another way, it may be described as what happens when cortisol runs amok in the human body. The primary symptom of Cushing's is rapid weight gain, particularly in the face and around the middle of the body. Considering that the excess fat stored around the middle of the body called visceral fat is so dangerous that it can cause type 2 diabetes, heart disease and even cancer, you get a sense of how dangerous exposure to excessive cortisol could be.

One of the ways that cortisol seems to cause rapid weight gain is that it causes us to make bad food choices. In a number of studies, stress has been shown to trigger an appetite for foods that are high in sugar and fat, typically described as "comfort foods." If you have an abundance of stress in your life, it is highly likely that cortisol is stimulating your appetite in this rather disastrous manner.

It may be that some people are at a greater risk for cortisol-related health problems than others. British researchers have demonstrated that the subjects in their study that reacted to stress with high cortisol levels in an experimental setting were more likely to eat in response to ordinary stressful events in their routine lives than low-cortisol responders. So, the question is, are you one of those people at greater risk for experiencing the negative health consequences of cortisol? Pay attention to your eating habits. If you tend to eat more when you are under stress then the answer might be, "Yes, you are at greater risk."

There might be a happy outcome for people at higher risk of elevated cortisol levels. We may find that going on the Greek Yogurt Diet and exercising regularly are going to have greater positive effects on people at risk than it will for others. This means that you may have even more to gain from this plan than the average person. So, start paying attention to how you respond to stress once you are on this diet. Are you eating less during times of stress when—at the same time—you have been eating lots of yogurt? If so, that would tend to indicate that this plan is working for you and that you are on the right track.

Eating yogurt should reduce your body's cortisol levels. This can have a number of effects. One such effect might be that you will enjoy a reduction in appetite. Specifically, your craving for foods that are high in fat and carbohydrates might drop significantly. It may also mean that you will almost immediately see a reduction of fat around the middle of your body. For example, one of my patients lost 10 inches from his waistline after just one year of following the Greek Yogurt Diet.

Once you have the ability to put your unhealthy appetites on hold, you can plan ahead and eat yogurt just before the time of day that you normally crave sweets, for instance. Imagine that at every night, at about 10 p.m., you suffered from an irresistible urge to eat ice cream or candy. The craving comes on like clock-work. What should you do? The solution would be simple. Every night at 9:30 p.m., consume 3-to-4 ounces of non-fat Greek yogurt. The usual desire to raid the fridge at 10 o'clock may be short-circuited by the alpha-lactalbumin found in yogurt.

Throughout this book, we will be looking at ways to lower cortisol levels. Yogurt is only one tool in the cortisol-lowering tool chest. Diet, exercise, relaxation and general lifestyle changes can all act in concert to reduce cortisol levels.

CHAPTER 4

GET CHOOSY WITH YOGURT

The Greek yogurt business is currently in a state of flux as some yogurt makers that stayed on the sidelines during the initial boom in Greek yogurt now scramble to make up for lost market share. Not everyone in the yogurt business anticipated the level of demand that currently exists for Greek yogurt. As manufacturers attempt to get one foot in the Greek yogurt door, they find that the highly specialized technology used to make Greek yogurt properly is very difficult to obtain.

A highly advanced machine used to make the best Greek yogurt, for instance, takes approximately one year from the date it is ordered until the date that it is delivered to the yogurt factory. As an alternative, some yogurt manufacturers have opted for inferior technology. Due to the importance of whey protein for weight loss, it is extremely important that you purchase yogurt that has been processed correctly so that its whey protein has remained intact to the greatest possible extent.

Unfortunately, it is not always easy to find out exactly what processes are used by a given brand or how much whey protein exists in a given product. Greek yogurt producers typically do not provide you with the exact amounts of whey protein that exist in their products. Perhaps with consumer demand for a higher whey protein content, yogurt manufacturers will begin to provide this information.

WHICH BRAND IS MR. RIGHT?

In contrast to the practices of many Greek yogurt makers that routinely strain out whey protein, companies like Chobani make whey protein content a priority. Chobani's products definitely stand out in the yogurt market. In addition to the company's focus on whey content, its products have a taste, texture and richness to them that make them feel truly decadent. Also, Chobani's flavored products contain fruits and other ingredients that tend to have exceptional nutritional value. It is no wonder that Chobani has become one of the best selling yogurt brands in America.

Chobani began in 2005 when Hamdi Ulukaya spotted an advertisement in the newspaper. At the time, he was running his own cheese company in Johnstown, which is located in upstate New York. The advertisement was for a Kraft yogurt-making plant in Columbus, N.Y.

Mr. Ulukaya was born in Turkey where yogurt is made in what we refer to as the Greek style. He knew that there was a niche in the market that desperately needed to be filled with the beloved yogurt that he had eaten while growing up in his country of origin. The very next day, he set out to buy the former Kraft facility and made sure to keep on as many Kraft employees as he could.

His purchase of the plant led him to create a yogurt company first called Agro Farma, Inc., which used the brand name Chobani. Chobani means shepherd in both Greek and Turkish. He later retitled Agro Farma in the name of the brand: Chobani.

In a talk given at a conference in 2013, Mr. Ulukaya stated that he did not know what to do next after purchasing the facility and hiring back its workers. In his quandary, he decided that he needed to do something and so he began by painting the walls of the facility. "It was through that simple act of painting the walls that we began to see what we wanted to do with the yogurt and how it should all work," said Ulukaya. "None of us did this before. None of us had a business degree, but during this journey, we found out what we were made of."

Mr. Ulukaya next hired a yogurt master. After a year and a half of trial and error, Ulukaya and his master yogurt maker had created what he considered to be the perfect cup of yogurt. Mr. Ulukaya's yogurt first found its way into grocery stores in 2007. The rest, as they say, is history, and most people credit Chobani with popularizing Greek yogurt in America.

The good news is that Chobani Greek Yogurt has gained so much popularity that it is available almost everywhere. You can find Chobani Greek yogurt, for instance, at grocery stores, pharmacy chains and even at convenience stores. Chobani features a store locator on its website to use as a resource. Remember to make sure that whatever brand of Greek yogurt you choose does not strain out the whey protein.

ONE "COOL" TRICK MAKES GREEK YOGURT DELICIOUS

Before opening up a container of Greek yogurt directly from the refrigerator, try putting your container into the freezer for a short period of time. You will not be leaving it in long enough to turn your yogurt into frozen yogurt. You will simply be putting it in long enough to slightly change the taste and consistency. You may find, for instance, that it makes your Greek yogurt feel more like a dessert. You can experiment to see exactly how much time you want to keep your Greek yogurt in the freezer. Ten minutes might be enough for you or you might want to leave it in there for just a bit longer. For a lot of people that otherwise prefer regular yogurt, the use of the freezer converts them into fans of Greek yogurt.

ALTERNATIVES TO GREEK YOGURT

There are a few alternatives to Greek yogurt that you may want to consider. For instance, feel free to use regular, non-fat or low-fat yogurt made from cow's milk in place of Greek yogurt wherever Greek yogurt is mentioned in this book. While Greek yogurt that retains its whey protein content may have advantages over regular yogurt, regular yogurt still has relatively high levels of whey protein and has been proven to promote weight loss. Regular yogurts also serve as attractive alternatives when there is either no Greek yogurt available or when the only Greek yogurt available offers little whey protein.

Another option is to eat regular non-fat or low-fat yogurt made from goat's milk. The type of whey protein that controls cortisol and promotes weight loss is called alpha-lactalbumin. It turns out that **goat's milk contains approximately twice as much alpha-lactalbumin as cow's milk**. Yogurt made from goat's milk is not as widely available as yogurt made from cow's milk. However, yogurt made from goat's milk may be found in many natural foods markets. Parenthetically, yogurt made from sheep's milk may also serve as a substitute for Greek yogurt, but it is difficult to find in most parts of the country.

Keep in mind that low-fat and non-fat goat's milk products may be hard to find even in natural foods markets because the equipment needed to produce reduced fat varieties is costly, and most goat milk producers are small family farms. Perhaps with increased consumer interest, non-fat and low-fat goat's milk products will become more widely available. The ideal development would be the production of a non-fat Greek yogurt made from goat's milk that preserves its whey protein content. In the meantime, consider discarding the top layer of goat's milk yogurt that forms in the cup as it mostly consists of fat.

For people that are lactose intolerant or allergic to yogurt, whey protein isolate can be consumed as another alternative (except that the powder may not serve as a substitute in recipes, of course). Ideally, you will find a powder that combines whey protein with casein protein in order to better replicate the composition of Greek yogurt. After all, casein is not without its merits. For one thing, it digests slowly, thus helping you to stave off hunger for long periods of time.

TOP OFF YOUR YOGURT

You may purchase yogurt that already contains fruit, or you can flavor your own yogurt (see the recipe for Greek Yogurt Paired Simply with Fruit in Section 5). Adding fruit serves multiple purposes. First, it increases the fiber content. Second, it makes the yogurt seem even more like a substantial meal than it does already. This is important because you want to make sure that you get a feeling of satisfaction and fullness from eating yogurt, especially if you are eating yogurt in place of a regular meal. It will help you stick to the Greek Yogurt Diet. Third, the fruit content enriches your diet with vitamins, antioxidants and flavonoids. Flavonoids are special nutrients manufactured by plants. They can engage in anti-allergic, anti-inflammatory and anti-microbial activities. They can even fight cancer. Eating fruit with your yogurt, therefore, has many advantages.

In addition to mixing in fruit, feel free to mix a little granola into your yogurt if you feel like you need the added crunch. While we generally discourage the eating of processed grains, if granola is making your experience of eating yogurt better, then eating yogurt with granola is an acceptable trade-off.

SECTION 2

LIVE LIKE A GENIUS

CHAPTER 1

THE HIDDEN BENEFITS OF EXERCISE

We know that many people have tried to make exercise a part of their lives in the past but gave up after a few weeks or months because the routine grew tiresome or they simply lost their motivation. Whatever your past experiences might have been, your attitude towards exercise is bound to change once you understand what a big role exercise can play in controlling the hormones that regulate hunger and control fat storage. In fact, exercise has numerous other benefits that you probably never knew existed. Let us now take a detailed look at basic types of exercise, as well as the benefits that you can gain from them.

IMPORTANT HEALTH ALERT

Consult with your physician before starting any new exercise program.

CARDIO TRAINING

Training to ride your bike at increasingly faster paces is an example of cardiovascular training. Cardiovascular training (or, cardio training) can be described as any activity that results in increased breathing and sustained activity of the cardiovascular system that goes beyond a mere burst of anaerobic energy (energy generated in the absence of oxygen). In response to cardio training, your muscles will become stronger, and you will use energy at the mitochondrial level (the level of the cell's "power plant") more efficiently. Your body will also get better at burning fat.

The key to cardio training is intensity. You want to hit a kind of Goldilocks zone: not too intense but just intense enough. Typically, this means getting your heart rate up to 70-80% of your maximum heart rate. Your maximum heart rate is a number that drops by one for each year that you are alive. To figure out your maximum heart rate, subtract your age from 220 beats per minute. Then, see if you can get your heart rate up to between 70% and 80% of that new number. For example, if you are 22 years old, that would mean your predicted maximum heart rate is 198, and you should train in the range of 138 to 158 beats per minute. If you are not in good condition, it may take a few weeks of cardio training before you will be able to exercise at the 70-to-80% range of intensity. But if you get into your own zone, even if it is not 70-to-80% of your expected maximum heart rate, keep training at that lower heart rate because your exercise program needs to be something that you can sustain over the long term.

You also want to choose aerobic activities that involve some kind of resistance that affects your lower body. Walking, hiking, jogging, running, rowing, climbing stairs, elliptical training, cycling, aquatic exercise and cross-country skiing require that your feet experience some form of resistance. When your feet experience this resistance, the resistance forces the large muscle groups in your lower body to work against it. This results in a greater chance of weight loss.

The intensity of your workout is extremely important. A study conducted at the Lawrence Berkeley National Laboratory in California looked at the effect of workout intensity on both weight loss and weight control by comparing thousands of runners to thousands of walkers over six years. The study was published in *Medicine & Science in Sports & Exercise* in April 2013.

In looking at adults with a body mass index in excess of 28 (classified as overweight), **runners experienced 90 percent greater weight loss than walkers**. Running proved more effective than walking both for losing weight and for preventing weight gain. For instance, take a woman of average height with a BMI in excess of 28. If she runs 3.2 miles a day, she can expect to lose 19 pounds over 6 years by running, but she can only expect to lose 9 pounds over 6 years by walking a total of 4.6 miles a day (which is a walk that will expend the same amount of energy as the 3.2-mile run).

Running also proved more efficient. Take the same woman from the previous example. She can expect to save time by running. The 3.2-mile run will take her 40 minutes to complete. In contrast, the 4.6-mile walk will take her one hour and twenty minutes. This means that walking took twice as long as running in order to expend the same amount of energy. Thus, you may be able to cut your exercise time in half by exercising vigorously.

The Lawrence Berkeley National Laboratory study demonstrates that any kind of intense cardio training, not just running, will give you more bang for your exercise buck because of the ability of intense cardio training to rev up your metabolism. Keep in mind that while you want to exercise intensely, you do not want your heart rate to go above 70-to-80% of your expected maximum heart rate.

While walking may not be the best form of cardio training, it should be emphasized that it is much better to walk than to get no exercise at all. If walking is your preferred form of cardio training, then walk at a brisk pace in order to maximize the benefits. Also, walk at an incline (up a hill or any steep grade) whenever possible in order to get even more from walking. Walking at an incline may be most easily achieved by using an inclined treadmill and attempting to walk at the highest elevation setting that is safe and comfortable for you. It should also be noted that walking works just as well as running when it comes to reducing heart disease risk factors such as high cholesterol, blood pressure and blood sugar levels, according to a study published online in *Arteriosclerosis, Thrombosis and Vascular Biology* in April 2013. When we say that running is superior to walking, we are not saying that walking has no value. It certainly does have value, and we encourage you to walk if more vigorous exercise is not possible for you at this time.

RESISTANCE TRAINING

Resistance training, or weight training, is a form of exercise that requires your muscles to alternately contract and expand in order to respond to some form of resistance. The goal of resistance training is to increase the level of resistance over time so that you attain specific physiological improvements in your lean body mass.

One improvement that you are seeking is hypertrophy (muscle enlargement). When your muscles start to enlarge, it means that you are seeing an increase in lean muscle mass. This increase in muscle mass is your body's way of coping with an increased intensity of resistance. More muscle mass is good for weight loss because it means that you will have more muscle tissue available to burn calories.

In order to achieve hypertrophy, you may use anything from calisthenics (such as push-ups and sit-ups) to yoga to rubber bands to free weights to weight-lifting machines. In order to maintain your current level of lean body mass, you will want to include at least 8 or 9 exercises so that you will be able to affect every major muscle group in your body. Your major muscle groups may be found in your calves, thighs, buttocks, abdomen, chest and arms.

Resistance training is highly encouraged. It offers a number of benefits for your health. It may increase the muscle mass being engaged by cardiovascular exercise. It may also increase your basal postural metabolism, revving up your ability to burn fat (although to a lesser degree than cardio training). Furthermore, resistance training appears to help delay the onset of Alzheimer's disease for the elderly. In addition, the chance of an elderly person falling can be reduced through resistance training by at least 30% due to improvements in poise, gait and balance. This is especially important because older adults are at greater risk for serious injuries—such as bone fractures—that can result from falling. Finally, strength training can be used to alleviate certain types of arthritis pain either in place of medication or as part of a treatment plan that includes medication. In light of the many health benefits attributed to resistance training, we strongly encourage you to incorporate resistance training into your overall health program.

CIRCUIT TRAINING

Rather than forcing yourself to choose between cardio training and resistance training, there is a type of exercise that comes fairly close to giving you the best of both worlds. It is called circuit training. It typically involves doing multiple exercises strung together into a predesigned "circuit." The exercises usually combine traditional cardio activities (like running on a treadmill) with resistance training (like push-ups). In order to make the resistance training portions of the circuit more like cardio training, resistance training movements are performed rapidly and then quick transitions are made from one activity to the next. While your heart rate will likely be lower when doing circuit training than it would be while engaging in pure cardio training, the benefits of resistance training should make it a worthwhile part of your exercise program.

OFF THE BEATEN PATH

For some people, traditional exercise will always feel like drudgery. If you need to do something besides running and cycling, here are a few surprising activities that may cause you to work up a sweat.

Hula hooping can burn 100 calories in just 10 minutes. Also, a half-hour game of darts can burn up to 100 calories. Jumping rope can burn up to 150 calories in just 10 minutes, and you may be able to burn up to 100 calories in 10 minutes by doing jumping jacks. Dancing can burn 200 calories in 35 minutes.

You may also consider taking a trip to the mall. Walking from shop to shop can burn up to 100 calories in 30 minutes. Also, each time you try on an outfit you may burn up to 10 calories for your efforts. Be sure to steer clear of cinnamon buns and other food traps while you are strolling.

On your way home from the mall, go grocery shopping. It is possible to burn up to 117 calories after just 45 minutes of pushing your cart around the supermarket. Then, once you get home, you can burn up to 40 additional calories unloading the groceries from your car into your house. You will burn even more calories if you need to climb stairs in order to get the job done. This means that a trip to the grocery store can burn off up to 157 calories or more.

Household chores might become more glorious once you learn that vigorous cleaning can burn up to 135 calories an hour. Mopping can burn up to 170 calories an hour, and bathing a dog while standing up can also burn up to 170 calories an hour. Painting a room may allow you to burn up to 200 calories an hour, and moving furniture can burn up to 400 calories an hour.

Even going to a movie can help you lose weight. Twenty minutes of raucous laughter while watching a comedy can burn up to 70 calories alone. Scary movies can help you burn even more. Researchers at the University of Westminster in England found that people can burn up to 184 calories by watching a single shocking horror film. Just make sure that you skip those fat-laden nachos when you pass the concession stand.

ADD TECHNOLOGY

Consider purchasing a Fitbit. The Fitbit is a full-featured pedometer that automatically keeps track of your steps, distance and calories burned. It also acts as a wellness monitor. A Fitbit can upload wirelessly to a web site in order to provide you with graphs and charts visually informing you of the number of steps that you have taken, the distance you have traversed and the quality of your sleep. It can also track your diet, heart rate, blood pressure and glucose levels.

The device is smaller than most pedometers and can be worn discreetly on a waistband or in a pocket. It works with both PC and Mac computers and charges no subscription fees for monitoring your activity online. Fitbit also offers an iPhone app and an Android app, and it works in concert with an increasing number of other apps and fitness tracking sites that have been developed in order to integrate seamlessly with Fitbit technology.

The Fitbit pedometer displays steps, distance, calories and a growing flower in order to visually display your progress as you work towards your daily goal. While it performs silently, you can upload your data to the Internet to be compiled in ongoing graphs and stats in order to show you if you are on track with your diet.

The Fitbit makes very few technical demands of its user. The pedometer has only one button, and it automatically resets each day. You may use it to measure sleep periods and sleep quality by simply pressing the button for a couple of seconds in order to start and stop that function. The Fitbit has no additional technical requirements.

Logging into Fitbit on your computer, you will see how many calories have been burned in five minute intervals, and each interval is color coded for intensity. It adds up steps taken, distance traveled and provides you with a so-called active score.

If you wear the unit to bed in its wristband or just clipped to your nightwear and remember to start and stop it in sleep mode, Fitbit will help you to track your sleep pattern. Fitbit provides you with a sleep efficiency score, tracks when you went to bed, tells you how many times you awakened during the night, informs you of how long you were in bed and gives you your total sleep time. The Fitbit is not a substitute for a proper sleep study, however, as it does not measure all aspects of your sleep and has no way of telling if you woke up briefly but immediately fell back to sleep without being conscious of the fact that you have awakened.

Fitbit also allows you to track your mood each day, record any allergic reactions that you have had and maintain any custom log that you may want to keep. You may, for instance, want to keep a log showing cigarettes smoked, alcoholic beverages consumed, strength training accomplished, stretching performed or anything else for that matter. You may also use Fitbit to keep a running journal about the events that occur each day.

Fitbit has a social networking aspect, as well. You and your friends may use a Fitbit to see how you compare with one another when it comes to steps taken, distance traveled and other aspects of your active day. You may also join groups and compare your performance with the performance of the group. All in all, a Fitbit may make a good investment for your health.

EXERCISE AND CORTISOL

As your cardio training improves, the amount of cortisol that your body produces in order to deal with stress may diminish. Remember that the body releases cortisol during times of stress? Cardio training can condition your body to manage greater levels of stress without resorting to cortisol. In order to illustrate this point, imagine that the fastest pace you can ride your bike is 20 mph. This means that whenever you hit the speed of 20 mph or higher, your body will release cortisol. But if you train harder and improve your speed so that you are now regularly getting up to 25 mph, your body may release less cortisol when you are only going, say, 20 mph.

Cardio training can improve your stamina and minimize the cortisol that your body releases in order to deal with stress in general. You may find that the benefits last beyond the time you spend in the gym. Studies show that when an individual who gets regular exercise has an emotional crisis, that person will have diminished cortisol levels compared to someone that does not exercise regularly.

It is not just formal exercise that can play this role in your body. A study compared cortisol levels in people that lead an active lifestyle to people that lead a sedentary lifestyle. It turns out that simply standing more, walking more and doing more leads to less cortisol being released in your body when compared to people that spend most of the day sitting around. So, get out of your chair and get active.

STIFLE YOUR APPETITE

Another benefit of cardio training is that it may actually suppress your appetite, and wouldn't we all like to have the ability to eat less without suffering from the pangs of hunger? Cardio training controls the entry of two critical appetite hormones into your bloodstream. The first hormone is ghrelin, the hormone that boosts appetite. The second hormone is peptide YY, the hormone produced in the digestive system that reduces appetite. In 2008, the journal *Regulatory Integrative and Comparative Physiology* published a study that compared subjects running on a treadmill, a form of cardio training, for 60 minutes to subjects engaged in resistance training for 60 minutes. The subjects running on a treadmill enjoyed a greater drop in hunger compared to the subjects in the control group that merely engaged in resistance training. When the scientists tested all of the subjects' ghrelin and peptide YY levels, they found that cardio training had simultaneously *lowered* ghrelin levels and *increased* peptide YY levels, resulting in a diminished appetite.

DURING AND AFTER

The next benefit of cardio training is that, during your conditioning, your body will burn calories and help you to slim down. The more you exercise, the more calories your body will burn. Then, after you stop exercising, the burn may continue.

According to a recent study in *Medicine & Science in Sports & Exercise*, a group of men that rode stationary bicycles for 45 minutes at 75-to-80% of their maximum heart rate (on average) used up 519 calories while they exercised, and then burned an additional 193 calories in the following 14 hours. They continued to burn calories due to the fact that their cardio training had revved up their metabolisms.

The key to burning calories after a workout is intensity. You must engage in vigorous exercise to reap the maximum benefits of an after-burn. Mere walking, for instance, will not lead to significant post-workout calorie burns. So, if you are capable of working out intensely, post-workout calorie burns provide an additional reason to exercise with vigor.

KEEP YOUR MUSCLE

Exercise not only help you to lose body fat. It also helps you to maintain your bone density and keep your lean body mass. There are two forms of exercise that can help you to achieve this result. The primary form of exercise for maintaining bone density and lean body mass is cardio training. The secondary form of exercise that we are going to look at is resistance training.

You should view cardio training as absolutely necessary for the purposes of maintaining both bone density and lean body mass. Resistance training, while helpful for our purposes, is not strictly necessary if you are getting adequate amounts of cardio training. The reason that cardio training is so effective is that it is systemic. This means that it affects a wide range of organs and tissues throughout the body, even improving tissues that are not directly involved in the cardiovascular activity. Resistance training, on the other hand, only affects those tissues that are involved, either directly or indirectly, in the specific resistance training activity. For these reasons, place your emphasis on cardio training.

MAINTENANCE IS A MUST

Cardio training is the key to maintaining weight loss. Studies show that the majority of people who manage to sustain their new weight for 12 full months following the end of their weight loss did so by exercising 60-to-90 minutes per day, each and every day of the week. The amount of exercise did not need to be severe. While intense exercise is ideal, moderate exercise proved to be adequate. This means that simply walking at a somewhat brisk pace for about an hour a day should do the job. The key is being consistent and making exercise a permanent part of your lifestyle.

To give you some idea of how important exercise is in maintaining the results obtained through dieting, consider what happens when successful dieters fail to exercise. Studies have shown that, despite being previously successful in losing weight, when subjects neglect to exercise, more than 90% of non-exercisers regain most or all of the weight they had previously lost by changing their eating habits. Some even gain more weight than they had originally lost. Unless you think that you will have more luck than 90% of successful dieters you must start to exercise now and never give up on it. Exercise is the pillar for maintaining your weight loss.

CATCH SOME Z'S

The last benefit of cardio training is that it can help you to achieve a regular sleep schedule. Sleep is a vital component of a winning weight-loss lifestyle. We discuss sleep in greater detail below in Chapter 3 of this section ("Sleep Your Way Thin"). When you slip into a proper sleep cycle, you should experience less of the hunger that would otherwise be brought on by sleep deprivation.

According to a recent study conducted at Northwestern University, cardio training appears to hold the key to treating insomnia, and it appears to work without the need for any medication. This gives us one more solid reason to enjoy cardio training on a regular basis.

Subjects in the experimental group exercised at 75% of their maximum heart rate while riding a stationary bicycle, walking, or exercising on a treadmill, and they did so four times a week.

The investigators reported that the subjects in the experimental group stated that their sleep experience was enhanced. They went from being rated as poor sleepers to being rated as good sleepers. Significantly, they experienced less depression, less fatigue and fewer incidents of sleepiness during waking hours.

CHAPTER 2

THE ZEN OF WEIGHT LOSS

The everyday stress in our lives can cause the release of the stress hormone called cortisol. As we have seen, excess amounts of cortisol can be severely damaging to our bodies and make it difficult to lose weight. Fortunately, there is more than one way to reduce our cortisol levels. In addition to exercising and consuming whey protein, we can reduce the amount of cortisol acting on our bodies through stress management.

There are several activities that will help you to manage your stress more effectively. At first, some of these activities might seem a bit silly. However, science confirms that the principles behind these techniques are sound. Find 10-to-20 minutes in the middle of a stressful day to go through one or more of the exercises below. But first, find a safe, quiet place where you will not be interrupted.

THE PRESENT MOMENT

A 2013 study conducted at the University of California at Davis Center for Mind and Brain published in *Health Psychology* showed that simply practicing mindfulness meditation can lower the levels of cortisol found in the body. Mindfulness meditation simply involves becoming deeply aware of the present moment. Sit or lie down. Relax your jaw and touch your tongue to the roof of your mouth. Your eyes may be closed or remain open, as you prefer. If you find yourself drifting off to sleep at any point, then keeping your eyes open during this exercise may be best. Next, draw slow, deep and regular breaths through your nose until you find that your breathing has fallen into a comfortable rhythm. As you slow your breathing, your heart rate will also begin to slow.

As you feel yourself start to relax, allow your present circumstances to draw in your focus. Let yourself become aware of the present moment without making any judgments about what you are experiencing or thinking. Simply bear witness and allow yourself to experience complete harmony with the positive aspects of your surroundings. You should begin to feel a greater sense of clarity and calm.

PROGRESSIVE MUSCLE RELAXATION

The Progressive Muscle Relaxation method allows you to reduce stress by alternately tensing and relaxing the muscles in your body. It was developed by an American physician named Edmund Jacobson in the early 1920s. Progressive muscle relaxation involves both a physical and a mental component.

The physical component involves alternately tensing and relaxing muscle groups in the legs, abdomen, chest, arms and face. When you tense your muscles, it should be subtle. You are not flexing them like a bodybuilder in an attempt to increase muscle mass. You are merely tensing them, without motion, and are doing so almost imperceptibly to others.

With the eyes closed and in a sequence that moves from one muscle group to the next, you purposefully tense up one muscle group for approximately 10 seconds, and then you release the tension for 20 seconds. At the end of the 20 seconds, you move to the next muscle group and tense up for 10 seconds, and the cycle continues.

You may begin by tensing your feet, and then relaxing your feet. You may repeat this by tensing and then relaxing your calves, then your thighs, then your abdomen, then your chest, then your arms and then the muscles in your face.

The mental component centers on noticing the difference between the alternating feelings of tension and relaxation. Because you have closed your eyes, the exercise forces you to focus on the way that tension and relaxation make you feel. Because a muscle feels warm and heavy after being tensed and relaxed, you will enjoy the mental relaxation that comes from the process and feel your stress simply melt away.

REVISIT HAPPIER TIMES

Think about one of your favorite days. Imagine that you have that day recorded on a DVD in your mind. Visualize putting that DVD inside of a DVD player within your imagination. Next, push play on the DVD player. Think about what happened in the course of that day. Imagine that you are reliving those experiences vividly. The sights, sounds and even aromas come back to you perfectly. Think about who was there with you and everything that you did that day. Remember how it felt. Remember all of the positive emotions that you experienced. Let yourself feel those emotions again, and let those feelings wash over you.

VISUALIZE THE IDEAL YOU

Imagine where you will be in five years. Imagine how healthy you will look once you have reached your goal weight. Visualize how good things will be. What goals do you want to see accomplished five years from today. Are they relationship goals? Are they career goals? Are they financial goals? Are they parenting goals? Imagine yourself achieving all of the goals that you have identified. Imagine how good it will feel to have accomplished what you set out to do. Let yourself bask in that sense of achievement for as long as possible.

EXPRESS YOUR GRATITUDE

Start a gratitude journal. Throughout the day, when something good happens to you, make a note about it in your journal. Take note of the positive things that people say to you and do for you. By placing emphasis on the good things in your life, the potentially stressful things that happen around you will cause you less stress. Build a core of happiness.

HEAT UP TO COOL DOWN

Physical exercise, as detailed in Chapter 1 of this section, can play a huge role in stress management. If you are feeling stressed out, then take a brisk walk for 30-to-45 minutes. Take the walk during your lunch break, if at all possible, in order to reduce your stress levels mid-day. If you do not want to engage in a cardiovascular activity because you do not want to get sweaty in the middle of your workday, try stretching exercises such as yoga. Or, take a walk at a more leisurely pace. Really, any kind of physical activity should help you to better manage the stress in your life.

GET A MASSAGE

An Australian study looked at a 20-minute massage therapy session offered daily to patients during their period of hospitalization. The scientists found a significant reduction in cortisol levels. The also observed a drop in resting heart rate and self-reported anxiety immediately following the massage therapy sessions. Do we also need to mention that massages feel great?

CHEW GUM

A 2008 study in Australia demonstrated that simply chewing gum reduced cortisol levels in subjects. Not only did their cortisol levels drop, the subjects chewing gum stated that they felt less stressed and experienced greater feelings of alertness.

Gum chewing has some obvious advantages. Unlike other methods of stress reduction, you can do it almost anywhere and at almost any time. If you are driving in stress-inducing traffic, for instance, you can pop a stick of gum into your mouth and continue down the road. You do not need to pull over to the side as you would need to do in order to practice mindfulness meditation. If you decide to chew gum, choose sugar-free gum in order to avoid calories and spikes in glucose levels.

HEALTH ALERT

Chewing gum excessively may cause health problems. Jaw muscles can become tired, possibly leading to pain and spasms. Gum chewing may even lead to TMJ, a painful condition that affects the ability of the jaws to function properly. So, be sure to limit your use of gum, and be sure to rely on other stress reducers.

CHAPTER 3

SLEEP YOUR WAY THIN

Sleep is an incredibly important component of a healthy lifestyle, especially if you are trying to lose weight. Not getting enough sleep on a regular basis can make you gain weight due to the effects of sleeplessness on four key hormones. Those hormones are ghrelin (pronounced GRELL-in), cortisol, peptide YY and leptin. Let us take a close look at how a lack of sleep affects each hormone.

Ghrelin is a naturally occurring hormone in our bodies that causes an increase in appetite. If you are trying to lose weight, then it is something that you will want to avoid. One of the factors that causes our ghrelin levels to shoot up is not getting enough sleep on a regular basis. Ghrelin gets out of control in the following type of scenario. Let's say that one night you go to bed at 11 p.m. and wake up at 6:00 a.m., and the next night you go to bed at 1 a.m. and wake up at 5:00 a.m. As a result of the inconsistency and lack of sleep, you will likely experience a spike in your ghrelin levels. With more ghrelin in your system, you will experience hunger pangs. The increase in appetite will lead you to eat more food than your body actually needs, possibly leading to obesity and other health problems over time.

But ghrelin is not the only hormone that you need to worry about. A lack of sleep can also lead to the release of the stress hormone called cortisol into your body. As we have learned, high cortisol levels can lead to cravings, overeating and bad food choices. The increased cortisol can even increase the storage of fat directly, especially into the middle of the body.

A lack of sleep also interrupts leptin activity. Leptin is a hormone that is made within fat cells, and it tells the brain when you have stored full reserves and no longer need to eat. If you fail to get enough sleep, your leptin levels will plummet. As a result, your brain never gets the signal that it is full and so the impulse to keep eating will continue.

In addition to a reduction in leptin production, a lack of sleep can interrupt peptide YY, the hormone produced in the gut that reduces appetite. Leptin and peptide YY work together to signal your brain to stop eating.

Simply put, if you do not get a minimum of 8 hours of sleep on a regular basis, it could have disastrous effects for your body. Shots of ghrelin and cortisol will tell your brain to keep eating. At the same time, a lack of leptin and peptide YY will prevent your brain from discovering that you are full.

To combat the chain of events that stems from lack of sleep, set a regular sleep schedule and make sure that you are generally getting at least 8 hours of sleep nightly. If you are having trouble sleeping, you should consult your physician. You may also try exercising regularly to improve your sleep schedule (see Chapter 1 of this section for a discussion on exercise and sleep). Below are some additional tips for getting enough sleep on a regular basis.

SLEEP TIPS

There are many steps that you can take to make falling asleep and staying asleep easier to achieve. We recommend that you develop an overall plan for getting a greater quantity and quality of sleep. Then, tinker around with various tricks to see what works best for you. Let us now share a few tips that will make a good night's rest more easily attainable.

You should generally avoid taking naps, especially later in the day. Save up all of your sleeping for one big block of time at night. Of course, if you absolutely must take a nap for some reason, then take one for the shortest amount of time possible. Set an alarm clock before taking the nap so that you do not sleep longer than intended.

Go to sleep at the same time each night and wake up at the same time each morning. Once your body falls into a regular sleep pattern, it will be easier for you to fall asleep and stay asleep all night. In order to wake up at the same time, it is helpful to use an alarm clock, even on the weekends.

If you snore or have apnea, then talk to your doctor. You might need a sleep test to determine if you would benefit from a CPAP machine or some other form of treatment. Once you lose weight, you may find that problems like snoring and apnea have become less of an issue, but you should get treatment for them in the meantime in order to address the immediate risks that they may pose to your health.

Check your room for noise or other distractions, such as street sounds coming in through an open window. If you cannot get rid of the noise, try wearing ear plugs or masking the sound with "white noise" generated by a humidifier, fan or other such device.

Do not gaze into sources of light for long periods of time close to bedtime. Sources of bright light that you should avoid may include televisions, laptops, cell phones and other electronic devices. It appears that sources of bright light may trick your brain into thinking it should stay alert as it would during the daytime.

Make sure that your alarm clock and other light sources are facing away from you while you are sleeping. Just a tiny amount of light may activate your pineal gland and stop you from reaching the deepest levels of sleep, such as REM sleep. Also, consider dressing the windows of your room with blackout curtains to keep light out or, as an alternative, simply wear a sleep mask over your eyes.

Keep your room temperature cool in order to make it comfortable to sleep under the covers. Sleeping under the covers improves sleep. In order to sleep under the covers without overheating may require the use of air conditioning during warmer months. If you sleep with a partner, make sure that each of you has his or her own blanket, as the case may be, because when a blanket is inadvertently pulled off of you by a partner it may make it difficult for you to get a good night's rest.

Avoid caffeine, nicotine and alcohol close to bedtime. Caffeine and nicotine may act as mild stimulants, robbing you of your sleep. Alcohol may be even more of a problem. Despite the myth that alcohol helps us to sleep better, alcohol consumption may actually cause sleep disorders by delaying the onset of sleep, disturbing the order and length of our sleep states and causing us to sleep less overall.

CHAPTER 4

ACTIVATE GOOD FAT CELLS

Do you remember the geese that laid golden eggs in the film Willy Wonka and the Chocolate Factory? Some of the eggs laid by the geese were "bad" and some of the eggs that they laid were "good." It turns out that while some of our fat cells might be labeled "bad" because they primarily store energy in the form of lipid droplets in order to create often unwanted fat tissue, some of our fat cells can actually help us to lose weight and should be labeled "good." The good fat cells are known as brown fat cells. When activated, brown fat cells actually burn fat. While the intended purpose of brown fat cells is to burn fat in order to keep us warm, we can harness the power of brown fat cells in order to lose weight. Physically, brown fat cells more closely resemble muscle cells than they resemble other kinds of fat cells, and they tend to cluster around the neck and collarbone.

It turns out that brown fat cells are more commonly found in women and thin people than in men and overweight people. Despite the level of brown fat tissue that you are born with, however, the good news is that it may be possible to actually convert white fat cells into brown fat cells. This means that the power of brown fat cells to burn fat holds out promise to all of us, even if we were born with relatively few brown fat cells.

The secret to converting white fat cells into brown fat cells lies in exercise. When you exercise, your levels of a hormone called irisin (pronounced EYE-riss-in) become elevated. Irisin exists as a component of a larger protein in the outer membranes of muscle cells, where irisin lays at rest within the larger protein like a bear hibernating in a cave. Irisin would remain dormant forever without something to act upon the larger protein, such as exercise. The act of exercising splits the larger protein apart, allowing irisin to break free and signal tissues throughout the body. Irisin is named after Iris, the Greek messenger goddess. Irisin is so named because it acts as a chemical messenger. When irisin encounters white fat cells, it appears to signal them to convert into brown fat cells.

HELPFUL HINT

It may turn out that irisin has other positive effects on the human body. When scientists injected small amounts of irisin into the muscles of animals that were both obese and showing signs of the lead-in to diabetes called pre-diabetes, the animals showed better control of blood sugar and insulin levels after just 10 days. This means that elevating your irisin levels through exercise may help you to stave off type 2 diabetes.

A pharmaceutical treatment for obesity based on irisin may someday be available. Alternatively, there might be pathways that do not involve irisin that will someday be used to convert white fat cells into brown fat cells (such as with BMP-7), or simply cause white fat cells to behave like brown fat cells. In the meantime, however, only exercise is available. If you want to maximize your body's ability to burn fat, then you may find exercise to be extremely powerful. Add irisin to your long list of reasons to hit the gym.

The main question when it comes to brown fat cells is this: How do we switch on the brown fat cells that we already have so that they go to work for us and burn fat? It turns out that there may be more than one way. In the future, substances such as the protein known as BMP-7 and the drug called amlexanox may gain FDA approval for weight loss. In the meantime, it appears that there are two ways to stimulate brown fat cell activity that are available now.

BMP-7

Some very exciting research focuses on finding a pharmaceutical approach to switching on brown fat cells. One promising avenue involves a protein called BMP-7. It appears as though BMP-7 not only switches on brown fat cells, it may turn white fat cells into brown fat cells. Scientists are currently examining how BMP-7 affects bone growth in human trials, which is an application that is unrelated to weight loss. In the same study that is investigating bone growth, researchers are conducting a preliminary study to see if BMP-7 is safe and effective for treating weight loss due to its apparent ability to activate brown fat cells and reduce appetite. In other words, they are piggy-backing the weight-loss study onto the bone growth study. If BMP-7 proves to be safe and effective in humans, then it could become available as a weight-loss treatment. As of this writing, however, BMP-7 has not been approved by the FDA for patients seeking to lose weight.

AMLEXANOX

A largely unknown medicine used to treat canker sores called amlexanox is another substance that appears to have the ability to cause weight loss. It does so by increasing metabolism. In an animal study conducted at the University of Michigan, subjects were first fed a high-fat diet and became obese. Some of the obese subjects were then given injections of amlexanox while others were not. The obese subjects receiving injections of amlexanox lost weight despite the fact that they were consuming exactly the same number of calories that they were fed previously. The control group that did not receive amlexanox did not lose weight. Like BMP-7, amlexanox has not yet been approved by the FDA to treat obesity.

COLD THERAPY

While BMP-7 and amlexanox are not currently available as treatments for obesity, it might already be possible to stimulate the activity of brown fat cells through one intervention that is readily available to most people: cold therapy. Researchers conducted a study in Sweden that was published in the *New England Journal of Medicine* in 2009. The scientists discovered that when people spent two hours intermittently dipping their feet into ice-cold water—five minutes on followed by five minutes off—while sitting in a chilly room, their brown fat went into action. They burned up to 15 times more energy than they did at room temperature. Some subjects had enough brown fat cells to lose several pounds per year at the calorie burn rate that they demonstrated in the study.

In addition to stimulating brown fat cells, cold can have other benefits. For instance, cold therapy has been shown to reduce pain in rheumatoid arthritis. Also, cold therapy increases glutathione (pronounced gloot-a-THIGH-own), which combats cancer, cardiovascular conditions, diabetes, inflammatory bowel diseases, lung diseases and osteoporosis. Glutathione is your body's own antioxidant, battling the effects of aging.

While we do not recommend spending two hours every day dipping your feet into ice-cold water (as the subjects in the study did), there might be some small things you can do to activate your brown fat cells while waiting for an effective pill to come on the market that will give you the same or better results than what cold therapy provides.

IMPORTANT HEALTH ALERT

Keep in mind that severe cold exposure can result in hypothermia and even death. You should only attempt cold therapy under your physician's supervision. While we recommend that you do your best to "stay cool," we do not want you to put your health in jeopardy by accidentally allowing yourself to suffer from exposure. This means that you should avoid immersion in cold water as exposure may result very quickly.

In the fall and winter, try keeping your house cool by not turning up the thermostat as high as you normally would. This will be good for both you and the environment. Also, wear lighter clothing both at home and when you are outside. Again, do not risk hypothermia by letting yourself get too cold. You simply want to be a bit cooler than you normally would be. For instance, if you typically wear a sweater under your coat, try wearing your coat without a sweater underneath. In other words, slightly under-dress for every occasion, if appropriate.

In the spring and summer, keep fans and air conditioners turned up. Also, wear lighter clothing than normal, if possible. Warm weather is the enemy of brown fat activity. In one study, animals that were fed a diet high in fat and kept at room temperature finished the experiment **weighing four times as**

much as animals that started out at the same weight and fed the same food but faced a constant temperature of only 39°F. The disparity in weight presumably resulted from the fact that the brown fat cells of the animals facing cool air burned off many calories as a way to create heat.

Most people do their utmost to winter in warm climates and summer in temperate climates. Instead, people should seek out cool temperatures year-round. Spend your winters in Vermont, Colorado or Lake Tahoe braving the cold. Ideally, you would spend your wintry days cross-country skiing or snowshoeing to get some cardio training while you enjoy the nice cold air.

In spring and fall, go on excursions that will get you outdoors to feel the cool air on your body. Exercise in the mornings and evenings when temperatures are at their coolest. Also, remember to under-dress for the occasion, as appropriate.

In summertime, spend time swimming. Or, better yet, spend some time in the southern hemisphere. June, July and August in Australia or Peru is actually their wintertime. If possible, head down to Sidney or Lima for your summertime fun. Alternatively, seek out the shore which is at ocean temperature (more or less) even in summer, provided that you keep out of direct sunlight. Boating provides purposeful activity at the shore, as do windsurfing, snorkeling, surfing and similar activities.

Exercising in cold air while wearing slightly lighter clothing may be extra helpful as it may allow you to enjoy synergistic effects. "Synergistic effects" means that you may achieve greater results by doing two or more things together rather than doing each at separate times. In other words, the whole may be more effective than the sum of its parts. In this case, combining exercise and the cold simultaneously may give you better results than what you would achieve by exercising in a warm room and then, at a later time, placing yourself in a cold environment. Therefore, exercise in the cold whenever possible to maximize both brown fat activation and muscle metabolism.

GREEN TEA

In addition to cold therapy, there is evidence that drinking green tea may activate brown fat cells. Scientists believe that the effectiveness of green tea is largely due to the presence of a flavonoid known as EGCG. In light of the effectiveness of green tea for making brown fat cells go to work for you, we recommend drinking green tea at various times throughout the day.

While you might be concerned about the presence of caffeine, green tea has natural relaxants that counteract some of the stimulant aspects of caffeine. Also, the caffeine levels of green tea are lower than the levels of many other caffeinated beverages. For instance, 8 fluid ounces of drip coffee contain 145 mg of caffeine. In comparison, 8 fluid ounces of green tea contain only 25 mg of caffeine.

In general, it is important to limit your consumption of caffeine because it can increase your body's cortisol levels. Also, it may act as a mild stimulant and keep you up at night. Unfortunately, decaffeinated green tea is not acceptable due to the fact that the decaffeination process destroys much of the flavonoid content of tea. However, you do not need to be overly concerned about the caffeine content of green tea because its caffeine levels are relatively minimal. Just to be on the safe side, though, it may be best to avoid drinking tea late at night in order to ensure that you are able to enjoy a good night's rest when you attempt to go to sleep.

SECTION 3

EAT LIKE A GENIUS

INTRODUCTION: A NUTRITIONAL STARTING POINT

The main purpose of this book is to show you how yogurt can improve your diet. However, before we talk about how yogurt can play a role in what you eat, let us first get a handle on what you should be eating when you are *not* eating yogurt. This will be your starting point. We have looked around the world and into human history in order to find the most optimal eating plans, and we have seamlessly integrated the best practices from multiple approaches in order to create the Greek Yogurt Diet.

We have provided the highlights of a number of approaches to eating: eating carbohydrates based on the glycemic index, enjoying the traditional cuisine of the Mediterranean, putting a modern twist on the food eaten by our distant ancestors, seeking out highly nutritious foods that we call "Genius Foods," eating and drinking to control cortisol, snacking properly and eating just the right amount of food with a special kind of awareness. Each of these elements has a number of important principles to teach us. We will put them together to shape an optimal diet for both weight loss and basic nutritional purposes. The Greek Yogurt Diet may not only help you to lose weight, it may also make you healthier in the process.

As a general rule, 10-to-35% of your total daily calories should come from protein, 45-to-65% of your total daily calories should come from complex carbohydrates and 20-to-35% of your total daily calories should come from fat. On the Greek Yogurt Diet, it is possible that the majority of your protein needs will be met by eating Greek yogurt. You will supplement the protein that you get from Greek yogurt by eating beans and other legumes, egg whites, skinless poultry, grass-fed beef, fish and seafood. To determine what you should eat to meet your carbohydrate needs, you should learn about the glycemic indexes of various type of carbohydrates and seek out complex carbohydrates in the form of fruits and vegetables. To meet your fat needs, we will help you to identify sources of bad fats to avoid and sources of good fats to consume. Because you will be eating a lot of non-fat Greek yogurt on this diet, it is important that you get enough good fat from sources other than yogurt.

Obviously, if you have food allergies or sensitivities, then you will want to omit those foods to which you are allergic or that you cannot tolerate. Likewise, if you are a vegetarian, you will want to remove meats from your version of the Greek Yogurt Diet. Your plan can be fully customized to meet your specific needs, either on your own or with the help of a dietitian.

We are not introducing yogurt to your diet just yet. Yogurt will be added later under the directions laid out in Section 4. As we introduce yogurt into your diet, the total number of calories and portion sizes that you consume will be reduced, allowing you to lose weight at a controlled rate.

CHAPTER 1

THE SMART CHART

A study by David Ludwig and his colleagues published in the *Journal of the American Medical Association* in June 2012 indicated that one's awareness of the glycemic index chart (and choosing to eat foods with a lower glycemic index) may prove far more important than one's concern over the number of grams of fat or carbohydrates that those foods contain. The scientists first compared low-carb, low-fat and low-glycemic diets to see which one burned the most calories per day. The low-carb diet burned the most. The low-fat diet burned the least.

However, a glycemic-index approach, despite only scoring mid-range marks for weight loss, might prove to be the best prescription. Not only did it burn more calories per day than the low-fat diet, it proved *easier for subjects to adhere to over the full length of the study* than did the low-carb diet. If you are looking for a principle that you can more easily follow until you have reached your goal weight, and for the rest of your life for maintenance purposes, then mastering the glycemic index of carbohydrates might turn out to be the best practice for you.

But first, what is meant by a glycemic index? Well, a glycemic index provides a measurement of how much the level of sugar in our blood (called glucose) increases when we eat a particular type of carbohydrate. An index is computed by giving pure glucose a rating of 100. In theory, all types of food are given a rating that should fall somewhere between 0 (for no change in blood sugar) and 100 (for the change in blood sugar caused by pure glucose). However, some types of food have a glycemic index that is greater than 100 for reasons that we will soon explain. The higher the index of a food or beverage, the more rapidly the carbohydrates in that food or beverage can be converted and absorbed into the bloodstream which is a process that you should seek to delay.

Considering that we should get between 45% and 65% of our daily calories from carbohydrates, the carbohydrates that we choose to eat will have a huge impact on our health. By using the glycemic index as a guide, we can be confident that we are making better choices about the majority of our total daily calories.

When we base a diet on the glycemic index of food, we do so with the understanding that a diet consisting of foods with a lower glycemic index will be more health-promoting than a diet made up of foods with a higher index. This is due to the fact that when the body suffers an onslaught of sugar in the bloodstream (which happens when we eat food with a high glycemic index) a chain of events is launched into motion. Let us take a close look at this dangerous chain of events.

First, your bloodstream delivers a sudden burst of energy in the form of glucose to your body. Next, your pancreas releases shots of insulin to regulate blood sugar levels and move the glucose into liver, muscle and fat tissues. Then, as your blood sugar level drops, you feel energy deficient, causing you to seek out more sources of sugar. Once you consume more sugar, your bloodstream will be loaded with glucose, and you will need more insulin. However, because your muscles are rarely exercised, they have become desensitized to insulin, forcing your pancreas to release even more insulin to compensate. Eventually, if you continue to eat more calories than you burn, this cycle will continue and your pancreas will not be able to produce enough insulin to clear the glucose. The less able you are to produce adequate levels of insulin, the closer you will come to developing serious chronic illnesses like obesity, heart disease and type 2 diabetes. This underscores the importance of choosing foods with a low glycemic index.

To give you an example of what a diet based on the glycemic indexes of foods would look like, it would emphasize eating foods like apples, which have a glycemic index of 39. You would avoid white bread which has a glycemic index of 101. By eating food with a lower glycemic index, you get less of a glucose rush in your bloodstream, and the chain of events described above that leads to diabetes and other diseases would be less likely to occur. Let us get more familiar with glycemic indexes by looking at the chart immediately below.

THE GLYCEMIC INDEX OF FOODS

Baked Goods	GI
Vanilla Cake	42
Banana Cake	47
Sponge Cake	66
Pound Cake	77
Danish	84
Muffin	88
Donut	108
Waffle	109

Beverages	GI
Tomato Juice	38
Soy Milk	43
Apple Juice (no sugar added)	44
Coca Cola®	63
Pineapple Juice	66
Fanta®, Orange	68
Cranberry juice cocktail	68

Breads	GI
Whole Wheat Tortillas	30
Coarse Barley Bread	34
Multigrain Bread	48
Whole Grain Bread	50
Oat Bran Bread	68
Mixed Grain Bread	69

Pumpernickel	71
White Pita	82
Hamburger Bun	87
Rye Flour Bread	92
Whole Wheat Bread	99
White Bread	101

Breakfast Cereals	**GI**
Rice Bran	27
Oatmeal (slow cooked)	55
Raisin Bran™	61
Muesli	66
Grapenuts™	75
Cornflakes™	93

Dairy Products	**GI**
Milk, skim	32
Yogurt with Fruit	33
Ice Cream (regular)	57

Fruit	**GI**
Grapefruit	25
Prunes	29
Pear	38
Apple	39
Orange	40
Peach	42
Grapes	59
Banana (ripened)	62
Raisins	64

Pineapple	66
Watermelon	72

Legumes	**GI**
Peanuts	7
Chickpeas (Garbanzo Beans)	10
Soy Beans	15
Kidney Beans	29
Lentils	29
Black Beans	30
Navy Beans	31
White Beans	31
Black-eye Peas	33
Baked Beans	40
Broad Beans (Fava Beans)	79

Pasta	**GI**
Spaghetti, protein enriched	27
Fettucini, egg	32
Spaghetti, wholemeal	42
Spaghetti, white	46
Macaroni	47
Macaroni and Cheese (Kraft)	64
Brown Rice Pasta	113

Vegetables	**GI**
Broccoli	15
Cauliflower	15
Eggplant	15
Carrots	35

Bell Peppers	40
Green Peas	51
Parsnips	52
Yam	54
Boiled White Potato	82
Instant Mashed Potato	87
Sweet Potato	70
Baked Russet Potato	111

Rices	**GI**
Uncle Ben's®, converted rice	38
Brown Rice	50
Quick-cooking White Rice	67
White Rice	89

Sugars	**GI**
Fructose	32
Honey	61
Lactose	65
High-fructose Corn Syrup	73

HELPFUL HINT

It makes good sense to familiarize yourself with the glycemic-index chart provided above so that you know how each food rates. Taking the time to familiarize yourself with the chart will pay off for you down the road in light of the fact that you will be making countless food choices over the course of a lifetime, and it will be tremendously helpful to have some guidance as you make those decisions.

FRUITS, VEGETABLES AND LEGUMES MAKE THE GRADE

If you are looking for foods with a low glycemic index, you would be hard pressed to do better than you can with fruits and vegetables. Nearly all vegetables have an extremely low glycemic index. While not included in the glycemic index table above, artichokes, asparagus, broccoli, cauliflower, celery, cucumber, eggplant, green beans, lettuce, peppers, spinach, squash, tomatoes and zucchini all boast a glycemic index that is below 50 and, in many cases, well below 50. If you are trying to follow a glycemic-index approach to your diet, then you will want to get most of your carbohydrates from vegetables.

The main exception to the rule that vegetables have low glycemic indexes is potatoes. A baked russet potato, for instance, has a glycemic index of approximately 111. This is unacceptably high. In fact, an index over 100 means that the carbohydrates in a baked russet potato enter the bloodstream faster than elemental glucose (sugar), which is used as the standard and has a glycemic index of 100. This happens because glucose molecules must get past cell walls one by one, but the straight chain of simple carbohydrates found in potatoes, flour, rice and other simple starches can be absorbed one entire strip at a time. So, it is easy to remember to avoid "white foods" when you remember how astronomically high their glycemic indexes are.

While not all varieties of potatoes have an index of 111, you should avoid eating excessive amounts of potatoes. Perhaps the only parts of potatoes that should be eaten freely are the skins, which contain approximately one-half of the total dietary fiber of a potato. The rest of the potato should be eaten sparingly. It should be noted, however, that potatoes, as whole plants, have much more potassium, fiber (complex carbohydrates) and protein than common flours comprised of milled grain starches.

Paradoxically, the much sweeter-tasting yam has a glycemic index of approximately 54, which is approximately half the glycemic index of the baked russet potato. This makes the yam an excellent substitute for a baked russet potato, even if it contradicts our intuition. Be careful, though. Once you start adding brown sugar to a yam, or worse, dress it with butter, you begin to undermine the dietary advantage.

When it comes to fruit, almost all whole fruits make excellent choices. Cherries, apples, dried apricots, pears, plums, peaches, grapes, oranges and kiwifruit all have relatively low glycemic indexes (below 60). They also have lots of fiber and flavonoids, the compounds produced by plants that are thought to be beneficial to our health. The exceptions to low-glycemic fruits are melons (especially watermelons) and raisins which have modestly high glycemic indexes. We should, there-fore, eat raisins and melons in moderation, focusing instead on the many fruits that have a lower glycemic index.

Almost all types of beans and other legumes have fantasti-cally low indexes. Hummus, made from garbanzo beans (or, chickpeas), is practically a miracle food. It has the low glycemic index of 10. But be careful about what you dip into it because pita bread suffers from having the relatively high glycemic index of 68. Choose, instead, to dip vegetables with low gly-cemic indexes into it. Carrots, broccoli and cauliflower are all excellent choices for dipping because they deliver a high fiber content and happen to taste delicious when paired with hum-mus. Be sure to eat it in moderation, though, because hummus does contain calories.

Another winner in the legume family is the peanut, gloat-ing of a glycemic index of 7. This makes peanuts an excellent snack food when eaten in moderation. Peanut butter is also acceptable, but make sure that you purchase a peanut butter with a low sugar content. Feel free to dip some celery or other vegetable into your peanut butter. Keep in mind that the por-tion of peanut butter that you should be eating is equal to no more than one tablespoon.

Green beans, snow peas, kidney beans, boiled lentils, gar-banzo beans and even baked beans all have extremely low glycemic indexes. The only kind of beans that you want to go out of your way to avoid are broad beans (or, fava beans), which top the list of glycemic indexes for legumes at a whopping 79.

You will note that, on average, fruits tend to have higher glycemic indexes than vegetables. This is because fruits tend to have more sugar, in the form of fructose, than vegetables. For this reason, we recommend that you emphasize vegetables in your diet over fruits. This is especially true if you are diabetic. Having said that, fruits are an excellent source of nutrition, and you should keep eating them. Just make sure that you keep a close eye on portion size.

DAIRY

Dairy products all tend to enjoy a relatively low glycemic index. The index starts to increase as we reach ice cream products. When we think about the total nutritional picture of dairy products (in addition to the glycemic index of each dairy product) keep in mind that not all dairy products are equal.

And on the subject of the glycemic index, there is some more good news about yogurt. Perhaps not surprisingly, low-fat yogurt has an index of about 14, which is extremely low. This furthers the excellent news that we have received about yogurt, and it informs us that following the Greek Yogurt Diet will also help to keep us on target with our glycemic-index goals.

PASTA LOOKS GOOD ON THE SURFACE

At first glance, pasta looks generally acceptable, at least from a glycemic-index standpoint. Protein-enriched spaghetti has the low index of 27. Egg fettuccini has an index of just 34. Pasta indexes are generally low due to the presence of branched chains in semolina wheat which means that a greater portion of the carbohydrates in pasta are complex. Semolina is also higher in protein than regular wheat.

Despite being acceptable from a glycemic index standpoint, however, pasta contains a significant amount of simple carbohydrates that fail to provide much nutritional value. Moreover, the fiber, proteins, minerals and other components of previously whole, living cells have been stripped away. Other than protein-enriched pasta, most pastas look a lot like empty calories, nutritionally speaking.

The goal is to minimize the amount of pasta that you eat to the greatest extent possible and opt for the healthiest options when you do eat pasta. For instance, choose protein-enriched pasta over non-enriched pasta. When you do eat pasta, we recommend Barilla PLUS® which contains pasta enriched with protein, Omega-3s and fiber.

AVOID MOST WHITE FOODS

White bread, white rice, baked goods, processed food and crackers all share one thing in common: They have a high glycemic index. Your body has the ability to break down these foods into sugar literally within moments of ingestion, even directly into the bloodstream through the tongue itself. So, in general, you will want to avoid most white-colored carbohydrates. The main exception to this rule would be most fruits and vegetables that have a white exterior or interior. For example, while cauliflower is white throughout, it is extremely good for your health and has a glycemic index rating of only 15.

THE PROBLEM WITH BREAD

Bread in any form is something to avoid or minimize, *even if it has a low glycemic index*. When you eat bread, your body will break it down into sugar in short order, and you will only obtain low levels of nutrients from it. As we will soon learn, bread was a health hazard as far back as ancient Egypt where it served as the cornerstone of the ancient Egyptian diet. Even then it caused hardening of the arteries that we can still see today in mummies. However, if you must eat bread out of convenience or for some other reason, at least seek out the more healthful options.

A few types of bread enjoy moderately acceptable glycemic-index levels. For instance, some types of multigrain bread have an index of 48. Whole *grain* bread (as opposed to whole wheat bread, which has been finely milled) can have an index as low as 50. To make sure that you are eating whole *grain* bread rather than whole *wheat* bread, look to make sure that either "whole grain" or "whole meal" is the very first item on the list of ingredients.

"Multigrain" simply means that the bread was made from more than one type of grain. If you are lucky, it may contain whole grains such as oats and whole grain. If you are unlucky, it may contain refined grains like whole wheat—or worse—white flour. Check the Nutrition Facts on the label. If it contains a minimum of 2-to-3 grams of fiber per serving, then it probably contains predominantly whole grains. Also, make sure that the ingredients list includes such items as whole wheat, oats, millet, brown rice or quinoa.

Whole wheat tortillas have the acceptable glycemic index of 30. You may use them to make a wrap. Or, better yet, use some lettuce leaves in place of whole wheat tortillas. Lettuce can make for a surprisingly delicious wrap due to the unique flavors and textures of the type of lettuce leaves that you use. We prefer to make wraps using butter lettuce (or, boston bibb lettuce). Their leaves are nice and thick. Also, they have a slightly sweet and buttery flavor. If you can eliminate or minimize the amount of bread in your diet, you will reap huge benefits.

HELPFUL HINT

If you must eat a sandwich for some reason, make it an open-face sandwich—using one slice of bread instead of two. Alternatively, have one-half of one sandwich (using a knife and fork if you need them), but pile high the fillings that would have gone into a whole sandwich into that one-half sandwich. Opting for an open-face sandwich or a "Dagwood" style half sandwich will cut in half the calories and sugar load that you would otherwise get from the bread.

SKIP HIGH-FRUCTOSE CORN SYRUP

High-fructose corn syrup is a sweetener made, as its name implies, from corn. It is composed of the sugar known as fructose. Like other sugars, fructose is completely nutrient-free. The high-fructose version has become America's sweetener of choice and is used in soda pop, candy and other processed foods. It is even used to make snacks, baked goods, cereals and soups. High-fructose corn syrup has a glycemic index of 73, but the number could vary according to the exact formulation of a given syrup.

In addition to looking at the glycemic index, you must look at the amount of sugar that the drink contains. A 12-ounce can of sugary cola typically contains 9 teaspoons of corn syrup. That is a ridiculously high volume of sugar.

New research indicates that high-fructose corn syrup is tied to obesity more closely than other types of sugar. Scientists at the Princeton Neuroscience Institute discovered that subjects consuming high-fructose corn syrup gained significantly more weight than subjects that consumed table sugar, despite the fact that both groups consumed the same total number of calories. Moreover, the group consuming high-fructose corn syrup over the long term suffered from increases in body fat, especially in the abdomen, and a rise in circulating blood fats called triglycerides.

In light of this new research, do yourself a favor. Pull your mouth away from that next "big gulp" of high-fructose cola, and have some water or tea instead.

NUMBERS CAN BE DECEPTIVE

Foods with a low glycemic index are not necessarily good for you. Many fried foods and high-fat foods that might seem like a good bet from their low glycemic index might actually be quite high in unhealthful fat. They might also be low in fiber, protein and other nutrients. You need to look at every aspect of what you put into your body, rather than considering only one factor.

For instance, Peanut M&M'S® have the relatively low glycemic index of 32. This is presumably due to the fact that peanuts, having the extremely low glycemic index of 15, offset the high glycemic index of the sugar found in the candy portion of Peanut M&M'S®. Obviously, the fact that Peanut M&M'S® have a relatively low glycemic index does not mean that you should make them the cornerstone of your diet. When you look at the nutrition facts label of Peanut M&M'S®, you see that they suffer from a high sugar content. So, be sure to look at every aspect of a food, not just at its glycemic index.

ADD FATS TO THE MIX

Take a look at a certain food that appears to have a relatively low glycemic index considering its category, namely, vanilla cake. Vanilla cake has the relatively low glycemic index of 42 despite being low in fiber and high in sugar. "How can this be?" you might ask. Vanilla cake has a low index solely because it is high in fat. Dietary fats cause the stomach to slow and retain simple carbohydrates. In fact, any simple carbohydrate can have a slower delivery of glucose when mixed with other foods that detain their digestion. This means that a food eaten during a meal will likely have a lower glycemic index than the same food eaten as a snack.

Beginning your meals with salad greens dressed with extra virgin olive oil will cause the stomach to close its outlet and digest its food for a longer time, releasing the calories more slowly. This will all be due to the fat content of the extra virgin olive oil. The glycemic index typically tests single-item foods eaten alone, and so it does not tell the whole story. Knowing that the composite meal will modify the release should allow you some latitude in composing your meals. And, appropriately, dark chocolate served at the end of the meal rides in the "caboose of the train." It is delayed in the stomach by the food that precedes it.

In contrast to dark chocolate eaten at the end of a meal, sugary fluids that you drink before and during the meal will run around and ahead of your food, quickly placing sugar into your bloodstream. Therefore, avoid juice and sugary soda drinks at all times of the day, even during your meals.

FIBER IS FANTASTIC

Dietary fiber, sometimes referred to as roughage, is the portion of plant foods that cannot be digested. By eating food that is high in fiber, you will ensure that the food you are eating has a low glycemic index. This is due to the fact that fiber delays the process of digestion and absorption in the gut. As a result, when you eat a high-fiber meal, the sugar content in your food trickles very slowly into your bloodstream. This slow-drip release keeps your blood sugar levels on an even keel and may prove vital for weight loss and disease prevention.

Eating fiber has a number of additional benefits. For one thing, fiber makes us feel fuller and gives us a feeling of having eaten something satisfying. One possible explanation of this phenomenon is that fiber stays intact inside the stomach, allowing it to take up more space and remain in the stomach for a longer period of time.

Due to the fact that fiber requires us to chew our food more rigorously, fiber makes eating take longer. It takes approximately twenty minutes after taking a bite before the stomach starts to send hormonal signals of fullness to your nervous system. Fiber buys you time. As you slowly chew your fiber-rich meal, you can get the message to stop eating before you have committed the "cardinal sin" of overeating.

Once in the stomach, fiber has a rather unique ability to make you feel fuller than you do with other types of food. It is the feeling of fullness that you get from consuming fiber that will make it easier for you to eat less than you normally would. For weight-loss purposes, this feeling of fullness can play a critical role in making your diet successful.

Finally, when fiber finally reaches the colon, bacteria begin to break it down. This is actually done through fermentation. This fermentation process yields organic acids that deliver an energy source for the entire body. Intriguingly, this fermentation process might also help to regulate your metabolism.

At this point, you should be excited about fiber and wondering how to get more of it. The answer is simple. Eat lots of whole fruits and whole vegetables, and you will get all of the fiber that you need. At the same time, you should avoid foods that have had the fiber processed out of them.

CHAPTER 2

THE MEDITERRANEAN MENU

Scientists have looked at what people around the world are eating, and how what they eat affects their health, in an attempt to discover the optimal diet. One of the best diets, and perhaps the very best diet for heart health, is based on what is eaten as part of traditional Mediterranean cultures that we like to call the Mediterranean Menu.

However, the traditional Mediterranean Menu may differ wildly from what people living in the region today might be eating. Exposure to the fast-food industry and other modern trends may have undermined the region's culinary traditions. For instance, fried foods have become much more common.

Whenever we refer to the Mediterranean Menu, therefore, we are speaking of the foods that have been eaten in the region for centuries and not necessarily what is eaten there now. The foods traditionally eaten on the Island of Crete represent a good example of such a diet. The life and health statistics of Crete are among the best in Europe even though Cretans do not enjoy high-tech medical advantages. Their wellness drives their health.

AVOID BAD FAT

The Mediterranean Menu is not low in fat, but it is extremely low in bad fats. There are two basic kinds of bad fat. The first kind of bad fat includes excessive consumption of most types of saturated fat. Most types of saturated fat are generally bad for us if eaten to excess. You should minimize the amount of saturated fat that you consume. The second type of bad fat includes Omega-6s. Let us first examine saturated fat in greater detail.

Saturated fat, in excess, appears to harm the cardiovascular system. A 2009 meta-analysis pooled the data from 11 studies that had been supported by the National Heart, Lung, and Blood Institute, National Institutes of Health, and other institutions. The meta-analysis found that substituting polyunsaturated fatty acids in place of saturated fatty acids resulted in a 13% decrease in coronary events, such as heart attacks, and a 26% decrease in coronary deaths.

While some studies have cast doubts on the extent to which saturated fats are more harmful than other types of fat, we think it best to minimize the amount of saturated fat in your diet until there is more evidence supporting the conclusion that saturated fat is no more harmful than other types of fat.

In the meantime, keep in mind that there is more than one type of saturated fat. Some types of saturated fat—like the stearic acid found in both beef and dark chocolate—are easily converted by our bodies into a healthful, monounsaturated fat. Thus, certain kinds of saturated fat, in moderation, might even be good for us.

The easiest way to eat the right kind of saturated fat is to include low-fat cuts of grass-fed meat from cattle or bison in your diet once or twice per week. In addition, we recommend that you eat up to 1-to-2 ounces of dark chocolate per day, which is an amount of chocolate about the size of your thumb tip. We recommend eating your dark chocolate at the end of your largest meal of the day in order to minimize the effects of its relatively high glycemic index.

The best way to minimize the potentially harmful types of saturated fat in your diet is to exclude foods containing lard, butter, cheese and cream (including sour cream) to the greatest extent possible. You should also make sure to remove the skin of the poultry that you consume. Finally, choose the low-fat or, ideally, non-fat versions of your favorite food items, such as yogurt.

IMPORTANT HEALTH ALERT

Be sure to avoid deep-fried food. Anything deep fried may not only contain saturated fat, it may also contain the very unhealthful trans-fatty acids (or, trans-fats). Trans-fatty acids simultaneously raise your bad cholesterol and lower your good cholesterol, giving you a double whammy from a single bad fat. Trans-fats may also be found in commercially baked goods (such as crackers, cookies, pie crusts and cakes) and even in shortenings and certain margarines.

Now that we have looked at saturated fat, let us examine Omega-6s. It is important to minimize the amount of Omega-6s in your diet for three reasons. First, Omega-6s are the precursor of arachadonic acid which results in a diet that can be inflammatory and harmful for your cardiovascular system, especially for women. Second, when eaten in conjunction with a high-carbohydrate diet, it appears that too much of these types of fatty acids can lead to obesity. In light of the fact that the goal of the Greek Yogurt Diet is weight loss, we consider Omega-6s to be counterproductive. Third, a diet that is too high in Omega-6s has been tied to arthritis.

Bear in mind that Omega-6s are essential fatty acids and that we need them in order to enjoy optimal health. The problem is that we consume far too much of them. The fact is that even if we did our best to avoid Omega-6s, they are so prevalent in the modern diet that it would be nearly impossible to avoid them entirely. Therefore, if we merely do our best to knock them out of our diet, then we will approach the right amount of Omega-6 fatty acids.

The main sources of the Omega-6s that we want to avoid are certain types of cooking oils and margarines. Sunflower oil, vegetable oil, corn oil, soybean oil, wheat germ oil, grapeseed oil and safflower oil are all chock full of the kinds of Omega-6s that we should seek to avoid. Other sources of Omega-6s include most types of mayonnaise and processed foods such as fast food and granola bars. Finally, avoid palm oil, palm kernel oil, peanut oil, coconut oil and corn oil.

The only exceptions to the list of vegetable oils that you should avoid are high-oleic sunflower oil and high-oleic safflower oil. They are both acceptable in moderation because they contain high levels of oleic acid (usually a minimum of 80%) which is the most healthful type of monounsaturated fat. In fact, it is the same type of fat that is found in extra virgin olive oil.

SEEK OUT GOOD FAT

There is a glaring misconception in popular belief that fat is bad for you. Many fad diets of the 1990s promised to make you skinny by cutting the fat out of your diet. What happened as a result was that people ate lots of simple carbohydrates that were easily turned into fat by the dieters' own bodies. It was a calamity that often caused people to gain rather than lose weight. The fat-free diet fad also failed to address the fact that fats play a vital role in good health and in helping us to lose weight. For one thing, fat slows digestion by delaying the release of sugar in the form of glucose into our bloodstream. This allows us to feel full for a longer period of time. In fact, the Center for Disease Control and the Mayo Clinic both want us to get up to 35% of our daily calories from fat in order to ensure that we are getting adequate amounts of health-promoting fat. The key is to eat the right kinds of fat.

The two best types of fat to eat are Omega-3s (polyunsaturated fats) and monounsaturated fats. Let us first examine Omega-3s because they offer a number of health benefits. For example, they play a key role in the construction of cell membranes. Consider the fact that cell membranes are 95% fat. If the body lacked fatty acids, then the body would not have cells. Also, Omega-3s keep the heart working by acting on the signaling membranes in cardiac cells. Omega-3s affect how cells interact with each other, and Omega-3s can even have an impact on how genes function.

Perhaps the most exciting reason to consume Omega-3s is that they may even help you to lose weight. Investigators at the University of South Australia Adelaide published a review in *Nutrients* in 2010 of the existing body of research that looked at the role that long-chain Omega-3s play in weight loss.

Most significantly, the researchers determined that long-chain Omega-3s work to suppress appetite. This means that it might make sense to consume your Omega-3s before meals. You may find that you will consume fewer calories as a result.

They also found evidence of improvements in blood circulation that they speculated might aid in the delivery of nutrients to skeletal muscle tissue. This improvement is responsible for burning more of the body's stores of fat. This indicates that there might be some benefit in taking Omega-3s before exercising in order to improve your athletic performance. Improved athletic performance may result in an increase in the numbers of calories burned.

They noted enhanced fat oxidation and energy expenditure. In other words, long-chain Omega-3s cause your body to break down larger fat molecules into smaller fat molecules and then burn away the smaller fat molecules. Omega-3s are like the 19th century engine-room workers that broke down coal and then shoveled it into the furnace so that it could be burned away into heat and smoke. Omega-3s help make the fat stored in your body disappear.

The researchers also noted reduced fat deposition. A reduction in fat deposition means that it was harder for the subjects to gain weight. Thus, long-chain Omega-3s may play a big role in helping you to maintain your weight loss once you have reached your target.

Intriguingly, the researchers also pointed to evidence that Omega-3s caused changes in gene expression that shifted the metabolism toward increased natural growth of lean tissue. This is important if you are trying to maintain or increase your lean muscle mass. Omega-3s may help you to grow muscle tissue.

You may obtain long-chain Omega-3s by eating salmon, halibut and tuna, as well as by consuming other forms of aquatic life that may contain Omega-3s to varying degrees. Flax, walnuts and soybeans contain short- and medium-chain Omega-3s that may be converted by your body into long-chain Omega-3s to some extent. And, as we will soon discuss, you may also supplement your dietary Omega-3s with molecularly distilled cod liver oil. The goal is to consume 4 times as many grams of Omega-3s as Omega-6s (a 4:1 ratio in favor of Omega-3s). Supplementation will make this goal much easier to achieve.

In addition to getting adequate levels of Omega-3s into our diet, we also need to get monounsaturated fat onto our plates. Perhaps the best way to consume enough monounsaturated fat is to eat "Genius Foods" (see Chapter 4 below) like avocados and almonds. By eating these Genius Foods, you will not only be getting monounsaturated fats into your body, you will be getting many other nutrients into your body, as well.

We can increase our intake of monounsaturated fat by opting for oils like extra-virgin olive oil and canola oil. We should also seek out margarines that name canola oil first on their list of ingredients. Instead of spreading such margarines onto bread, we recommend putting canola-based margarine onto cooked vegetables.

As we have learned, we may also cook with high-oleic sunflower oil and high-oleic safflower oil which are both acceptable in moderation because they contain high levels of oleic acid (usually a minimum of 80%). Oleic acid is the most healthful type of monounsaturated fat. In fact, oleic acid is the same type of fat that is found in extra virgin olive oil.

EAT MORE FRUITS AND VEGETABLES

A recurring theme of this book is that you should aim for a minimum of 4 or 5 servings of fruits and vegetables per day (assuming a daily caloric intake in the 1,600-to-1,700 range). There are some fruits and vegetables to avoid, as we have already discussed. Watermelon and the flesh of potatoes, for instance, have relatively high glycemic indexes. Eat them in moderation in the context of a meal if you cannot avoid them. You are encouraged to eat more than 5 servings of fruit and vegetables per day, but you should make sure to take into account the extra calories that you will be consuming and how they will affect your daily caloric intake of 1,600 if you are a woman or 1,700 if you are a man. See Section 4 for a discussion of the daily caloric intake that you will be aiming for while you are dieting.

Generally, fruits and vegetables have so much water and bulk per calorie that they help us fill up better than the concentrated calories of starch and meat. When you are trying to lose weight, fruits and vegetables should play a central role in your diet.

HELPFUL HINT

In order to get a wide variety of the special nutrients found in fruits and vegetables, pay attention to the color of the fruits and vegetables that you are eating. The reason is that the color of a food can alert you to the presence of one or more special nutrients found in that particular food. For instance, the color red may indicate the presence of the antioxidant known as lycopene (pronounced LIKE-oh-peen). Lycopene has anti-inflammatory effects, protects our skin from sun damage, gives us vigor in old age, decreases cancer risks and improves the health of our cardiovascular systems. We recommend that you eat fruits and vegetables that have as many different colors as possible throughout your day. There are five different categories of colors: red (example: tomato), purple (example: eggplant), orange (example: pumpkin), yellow (example: mango) and green (example: broccoli). A good goal is to eat at least one example of each of the five color groups every single day.

When selecting foods from the Mediterranean Menu, be sure to also seek out legumes and nuts as they help to comprise the traditional diet of the Mediterranean. Bean soups, for instance, have long been a staple of the Mediterranean Menu (see the recipe for Mediterranean White Bean and Kale Soup in Section 6).

OF FISH AND ARCHAEOLOGY

In August 2, 2002, members of a joint U.S.-Bulgarian research expedition discovered a shipwrecked, ancient Greek vessel off the coast of Bulgaria in the Black Sea. The team dove to a target that had been previously indicated by sonar in a three-person submersible vehicle launched from the 180-foot Bulgarian research ship *Akademik*. Twenty-to-thirty ancient pottery jars known as amphorae could be seen at the wreck site, but only one amphora was found intact. The jar contained olive pits, resin and catfish bones. Radiocarbon dating placed the catfish bones between the 5th and 3rd century B.C.

Cut marks appearing in the fish bones, together with other physical clues and knowledge of the era, prompted scientists to speculate that the amphora carried fish steaks. In the context of ancient times, this means that the catfish bones most likely came from two-to-three inch chunks of fish steak.

The archeological evidence relating to fishing in ancient Greek and Roman times includes fishing equipment, fish remains, fish processing facilities, transportation equipment, descriptive sources such as coins and paintings. It is important to keep in mind that, in the absence of modern refrigeration, fresh fish had to be consumed within 1-to-3 days of being caught.

At the same time, fish might have been preserved by salting, smoking, drying or being made into fish sauce. The fish sauce known as *garum* served as a key factor in the Roman economy. Consisting of fermented fish scraps in brine, *garum* was considered the taste of Rome and was imported by peoples living as far away as the outer reaches of the empire. Production seems to have reached its apex at fishing processing facilities around the 1st century A.D., but some *garum* producing facilities continued to operate as late as the 6th century A.D.

As you can see, fish and seafood have served as staples of the local Mediterranean diet and have helped to form an important part of the culture for millennia. From our perspective, fish and seafood are high in protein and low in harmful fat. Also, among the fats that they do contain are the highly beneficial Omega-3s, to varying degrees.

While fish and seafood should be a part of your diet, we recommend that you avoid eating fish that has been exposed to environmental contaminants and seek out fish that is environmentally sustainable. Fish that are high in omega-3s, low in environmental contaminants and eco-friendly include wild salmon from Alaska, Arctic char, Atlantic mackerel, sardines, sablefish, anchovies, farmed rainbow trout and albacore tuna from the U.S. and Canada.

While fish and seafood are highly recommended due to a number of their virtuous attributes, if you decide that you do not want to eat a diet high in fish and seafood, you may take molecularly distilled Omega-3 supplements instead. Taking supplements may help you to minimize your consumption of such contaminants as the heavy metals often found in fish.

Even if you are eating lots of fish and seafood, it is still a good idea to augment the Omega-3s in your diet with long-chain Omega-3 fatty acid supplements in order to ensure that you are getting adequate levels of the health promoting substances.

IMPORTANT HEALTH ALERT

Avoid canned fish. Canning boosts the amount of oxidized cholesterol in fish, particularly a molecule called 25-hydroxycholesterol (pronounced high-drox-ee-kol-EST-er-all), that poses an extreme hazard to the linings of our arterial blood vessels. This compound is so devastating that only 0.3% of our dietary cholesterol must be oxidized in order to cause untimely destruction to the arterial linings of our cardiovascular system.

CHAPTER 3

THE PALEO MENU

To understand the concept behind the 'Paleo' Menu, we must look back in time to about 20,000 years ago during the Paleolithic Era. The Paleo concept recognizes that we have come incredibly far as a species in terms of civilization and technological advancement over the past 20,000 years. The Paleo view is that despite outward advancements we are not much different genetically from our ancient ancestors. And because our bodies have only evolved enough to accommodate the diet that our ancestors were eating 20,000 years ago (due to the fact that evolution is a relatively slow process), our bodies might be ill-equipped to consume certain staples of the modern, post-agricultural diet. The basic hypothesis of the Paleo Menu is that by turning back the clock to look at what your ancestors were eating 20,000 years ago, or at least to some time before the start of agriculture, you will find clues about what an optimal diet should look like for a *Homo sapien* like us.

THEY MOSTLY ATE PLANTS

Let us revisit our recurring theme. A prominent goal in our Greek Yogurt Diet is to consume a minimum of 4-to-5 servings of fruit and vegetables every day of the week. This is based on a total caloric intake of 1,600 calories if you are a woman and 1,700 calories if you are a man, while you are attempting to lose weight. It turns out, coincidentally, that fruits, nuts and vegetables were the types of foods eaten in the Stone Age by hunter-gatherers. Of course, there was probably a broad range among hunter-gatherer groups, with some groups finding game to eat far more frequently than other groups.

Interestingly, it is believed that Paleo people devoured so much vegetation that they consumed between 100 and 150 grams of fiber per day. We are not asking you to replicate this achievement, however, especially in light of the fact that much of the fiber that our Paleo ancestors ate came in the form of woody stems and roots, stripped bark, and pith—all of which are terrible for your teeth and none of which tastes very good. We can guarantee you that we will not be seeing any of those items on a restaurant menu anytime soon.

Still, those ancient foods point us towards eating the high-fiber foods found in the fruit, vegetable and legume category in order to achieve optimal health. Thus, we may modernize the diet that our ancestors ate without compromising on fundamental nutrition.

FREE-RANGE POULTRY AND EGG WHITES

Free-range poultry tends to be more healthful than caged poultry, and it is the more ethical choice for you to make. From a health perspective, when birds are allowed to feed on greens (which contain the beneficial alpha linolenic acid) instead of grain feeds (which are high in omega-6s and void of the vitamins, nitrates and enzymes found in fresh greens) the meat will have a much better fat profile: more Omega-3s and fewer Omega-6s.

Of all the poultry that you can eat, free-range, skinless turkey breast might be one of the best food choices you will ever make simply due to its leanness. A 3-ounce serving of boneless, skinless turkey breast contains 90 calories with only 10 of those calories coming from fat. Turkey is also loaded with Vitamins B-3, B-6 and B-12, not to mention selenium and zinc. This dazzling array of vitamins and minerals can lower your risk for heart disease and cancer, and it can all be found in the humble turkey.

While turkey is generally healthful, be wary of highly processed turkey products as they can be nutritionally unsound. The turkey "bacon" you buy at the supermarket may contain much more sodium than even regular bacon contains, for instance. Meanwhile, turkey burgers are notorious for carrying traces of *E. coli* and drug-resistant *Salmonella*. In general, it is best to steer clear of processed turkey meat.

Chicken and duck meats can be good choices, but they tend to be somewhat higher in fat than turkey meat. Regardless of the kind of poultry that you eat, the key is to remove and discard the skin before eating it in order to minimize the amount of fat that you consume.

We also recommend eating egg whites as a good source of protein. Egg whites can be used in place of whole eggs by simply using two egg whites for every one egg specified by a recipe. Alternatively, a commercial egg substitute may be used in place of whole eggs. Read the label of your egg substitute in order to learn the equivalencies. Typically, one whole egg can be replaced with 1/4 cup egg substitute.

IMPORTANT HEALTH ALERT

We do not recommend eating egg yolks at this time due to their lecithin content. A study published in the *New England Journal of Medicine* on April 24, 2013, reported that lecithin may be linked to an increased risk of heart attack and stroke. This happens when the body breaks down lecithin into choline, and intestinal bacteria then metabolize choline. A byproduct of this metabolization is transformed by the liver into a chemical known as TMAO. High levels of TMAO in the blood are linked to an increased risk of heart attack and stroke. We, therefore, advise you to skip yolks until science sorts out this particular issue.

GRASS-FED BEEF AND BISON MEAT

It is clear that our ancestors hunted. Scientists now think, however, that meat provided a relatively small portion of their total daily calories. So, the idea is to eat red meat only once or twice per week. In order to try to replicate the diet of our evolutionary ancestors, we want to consume meat that has fed on a diet similar to what the game that our ancestors ate. For cattle and bison, such a diet would consist almost entirely of grass. In contrast to the ideal, most livestock in modern industrialized societies typically feeds on some kind of grain.

Grass feeding leads to beef that is much less fatty. For instance, a sirloin steak from grass-fed cattle has approximately one-half to one-third the amount of fat that a sirloin steak from grain-fed cattle contains. Amazingly, grass-fed beef has nearly the same amount of fat as skinless chicken or venison. When meat is that lean, it actually lowers your harmful LDL cholesterol levels when you eat it.

Another reason to eat livestock fed on grass instead of grain-fed livestock is that the fat profiles of livestock are improved when they are allowed to feed on grass. This means that ranchers feeding cattle grass produce a beef containing high levels of Omega-3s while the beef produced by a diet of feed grains contains high levels of Omega-6s.

When choosing a cut of beef, we recommend sirloin steak. Pound for pound, sirloin contains less fat and more protein than rib eye or porterhouse. Other lean cuts of beef include round steak, 95% lean ground beef and New York strip steak. Rounding out the list of lean cuts of beef are brisket and flank steak.

IMPORTANT HEALTH ALERT

You should limit the amount of red meat that you eat, even in the case of grass-fed beef. You should also avoid energy drinks containing carnitine. Research published in *Nature Medicine* in April 2013 indicates that the carnitine found in red meat and energy drinks may cultivate certain bacteria in the gut that, in turn, produce a chemical called TMAO. This is the same TMAO that results from the ingestion of egg yolks. When TMAO gets into the bloodstream, it increases the risk of heart disease and stroke. Our distant ancestors were lucky if they were able to eat red meat once or twice per week. We should, therefore, limit our own intake of red meat to no more than once or twice per week.

GOVERN YOUR GRAINS

Twenty thousand years ago, wheat was not a part of the human diet, and rice did not exist in plentiful supply. Both high-starch grains are relatively recent agricultural developments. In keeping with the Paleo Menu, wheat, wheat products, rice and other grains should be minimized due to the fact that our bodies have not properly adapted for them.

At the same time, you do not need to eliminate grains entirely in order to be consistent with the Paleo Menu. We simply want you to opt for fiber-rich vegetables over starchy grains whenever possible, minimize the total amount of grains that you eat and seek out whole grains instead of overly processed versions of those grains.

It turns out that starches are not entirely novel to humans. For millions of years, one of our direct ancestors, *Homo ergaster* (also known as African *Homo erectus*), survived to some extent by eating starchy tubers. Paleontologists also believe that the diet of *Homo ergaster* consisted in part of honey which mostly consists of simple sugar.

In light of what *Home ergaster* consumed, it appears that we may have evolved to eat simple carbohydrates, after all. It is simply a question of what consumption level is appropriate for us. By looking at health problems throughout human history, we can see that too many simple carbohydrates can still be hazardous for us. This is because they may be hazardous for us in large quantities despite the fact that we may have evolved to eat them in smaller quantities.

While bread is a more recent development than tubers, it did exist as far back as ancient Egypt and served as the principal food of the ancient Egyptians. This can give us a lot of insight into the health effects of refined grains. When we look at the MRI scans of mummies from ancient Egypt, we see that the Egyptians of that time period suffered from atherosclerosis (also known as hardening of the arteries) and showed signs of diabetes. Obviously, we cannot blame their diseases on fast food or processed food in light of the fact that such "modern marvels" had not yet been invented.

Many scientists theorize that the component of the diet consumed by ancient Egyptians that would have caused the hardening of their arteries was none other than the bread that served as the cornerstone of their diet. Keep in mind that ancient Egyptians did not have the highly processed wheat that we have today. In fact, they had the kind of bread that would have an impressively low glycemic index. Yet, even if it did measure up as one of the more healthful versions of bread that has ever existed, it still had terrible health consequences when eaten excessively.

The problem with wheat—and the problem with rice and other grains for that matter—is that the calories that those foods contain could, for the most part, be described as empty calories (using a somewhat broader definition of the term than the one provided by the U.S. Department of Agriculture). In other words, they offer relatively little protein or fiber. They are starches that dump glucose (sugar) into your bloodstream in short order. In most instances, when you eat a slice of bread you might as well be eating candy out of a jar. The nutrient profiles are that similar.

AN IMPORTANT NOTE

A gluten-free craze has swept the nation. Gluten is a protein found in wheat and other grains, such as barley and rye. People have been told about how damaging gluten is, and it can be for some people. However, it is only especially hazardous for a tiny percentage of the population, such as people diagnosed with celiac disease. For the rest of us, gluten may only be somewhat more damaging than the remaining portion of wheat. As a result of the gluten-free trend, many suffer from the false impression that they can continue eating gluten-free grain products simply because that specific protein has been removed. Unfortunately, what mostly remains when gluten is removed are simple carbohydrates that will cause considerable harm. In many cases, gluten-free products are nothing more than glorified junk food. Therefore, everyone except people with gluten vulnerabilities should avoid gluten-free products due to the fact that grains, in their totality, are bad for your health when eaten in excess. One particular protein is not our only worry.

We should also minimize our consumption of all manifestations of wheat. Various incarnations of wheat include orzo, semolina, faro, couscous, rusk, graham, panko, bran and matzoh. Just because something does not appear to be wheat does not necessarily make it something other than wheat. It may simply be wheat in disguise.

We should also minimize our consumption of grains other than wheat such as white rice, brown rice and wild rice. Your consumption of additional grains like rye, oats, bulgur, quinoa, amaranth, barley, millet, sorghum, spelt and buckwheat should also be reduced. Finally, your consumption of vegetables that have a nutrient profile similar to grains, such as corn and the flesh inside of potatoes, should be minimized.

Ultimately, we should minimize our consumption of all forms of grain products, especially highly processed grain products. These forms include bread, wraps, tortillas, pasta, cakes, cookies, pies, pancakes, waffles and breakfast cereals. It may prove difficult for you to cut back on many of these items. Although you may have grown accustomed to them, your weight-loss goals will be far easier to achieve if you can surrender your attachment to such foods and opt for more healthful alternatives whenever possible.

In place of grain flours, try cooking with flours made from garbanzo beans, almonds and coconuts. In the case of almond flour, for instance, one-half cup of almond meal contains 10 grams of protein, 6 grams of fiber and only 4 grams of simple carbohydrates. It provides an immediate improvement over wheat flour. You can find such flours in natural foods store and use them to make everything from pretzels to biscuits to pie crusts.

When you do eat grains, make sure that you are eating whole grains only. By eating whole grains in place of processed grains, you may even discover that you are taking inches off your waistline. A study published in *The American Journal of Clin-*

ical Nutrition in 2008 showed that a restricted calorie diet rich in whole grains had a powerful effect on belly fat. The people who ate whole grains, but no processed grains (in addition to eating five servings of fruits and vegetables, three servings of low-fat dairy, and two servings of lean meat, fish, or poultry), lost more weight from the abdominal area than another group that ate the same diet but also ate refined grains instead of whole grains. One example of an excellent whole grain is steel-cut oats. See our recipe for Pumpkin Oatmeal with Greek Yogurt in Section 5.

SHUN EMPTY CALORIES

As you might have guessed, empty calories were fairly hard to come by 20,000 years ago. Back then, the "sweet tooth" that all humans share attracted our ancestors to ripe fruits that were loaded with nutrients. Modern-day confections like jelly beans and cupcakes were not even dreamt of by our distant ancestors. So, to follow the Paleo Menu faithfully, we should do our best to avoid empty calories. Our bodies are simply not equipped to deal with them, and they tend to cause a number of health problems.

The U.S. Department of Agriculture (USDA) defines empty calories as calories obtained from solid fats and added sugars (which the USDA describes as food components that provide little nutritional value). "Added sugars" refer to caloric sweeteners put into foods during processing and show up on ingredient lists as sugar, corn sweetener, syrup, corn syrup, high-fructose corn syrup, fruit juice concentrates, fructose, dextrose, glucose, lactose, maltose, sucrose, and molasses. Honey also counts as an added sugar, but it at least offers some health benefits. Also, it appears that at least one of our distant ancestors, *Homo ergaster*, made honey part of his diet. Empty calories should be minimized to the greatest extent possible, however, even honey.

You might be wondering exactly what you can do to avoid empty calories. Before you eat something, ask yourself a simple question: Did our ancestors living 20,000 years ago eat what you are about to put in your mouth? If the answer is no, then you should probably avoid eating it or eat it only on rare occasions. Did they have cola sodas 20,000 years ago? No. Did they have cake? No. Did they have ranch-flavored tortilla chips? No. Did they have lemon meringue pie? No. Did they have bread? No. Did they have frozen caramel coffee drinks? No, again. And while it might seem a bit severe to avoid so much of modern food and drink, you will be doing yourself a huge favor if you can find the strength to say, "No."

DON'T GET JUICED

I once treated a diabetic patient with an alarmingly high blood-glucose level—over 700. Previously, she had generally been in control, meaning that she did not requiring insulin. She had always been one of my favorite patients and had a charming personality. I asked her, "So, what exactly have you been doing differently or eating differently now, with your blood sugar so high?"

She replied, "I'm not eating candy, Dr. Guetzkow. I'm not drinking soda. I'm not doing anything like that—I'm just eating normal food. That's it. Oh, and I drink about a gallon of apple juice every day. But it says 'No Sugar Added' on the label so that can't be the cause."

Bingo! Apple juice has an incredibly high amount of sugar—in the form of fructose—which is readily converted by the human body into blood sugar, glucose. It needs no added sugar because it already has plenty of its own. Drinking a gallon of apple juice is not equivalent to eating a bunch of apples. In fact, almost all types of juice have this problem. You are getting the sugars of the fruit or vegetable that you are eating, and you are missing out on most of the good stuff.

It turns out that juice is a hidden source of empty calories (if we use a definition of empty calories that is broader than the U.S. Department of Agriculture's definition). We assume that, due to their healthful origins as whole fruits or whole vegetables, fruit juices or vegetable juices will be equally sound nutritionally. We might even think that we are meeting our daily fruit and vegetable needs by drinking juice. The problem is that the juicing process strips away the fiber and other nutrients contained in whole fruit. What remains, in the case of most fruit juice, is sugar water with only a tiny residue of good things such as vitamins, minerals and flavors. In short, most of what makes up fruit juice might be described as empty calories.

In contrast to juice, eating whole fruits delays the breaking down of millions of cellulose and hexose cell walls which, in turn, delays the release of a fruit's juice. It makes a difference. You get less of a glucose rush and more fiber. You also get a longer lasting and more satisfying sense of fullness.

Not surprisingly, juice was not on the menu 20,000 years ago. Our ancestors ate whole fruits. Not only are fruit juice and vegetable juice inconsistent with the Paleo Menu, most mainstream nutritionists recommend that you avoid drinking juice in any quantity. In the case of fruit, you should either eat it whole or, if you must drink it, put pieces of fruit into a blender to make a smoothie rather than just press off the watery part. Obviously, smoothies were not an option 20,000 years ago, but blenders do little to alter the nutrient profiles of our favorite fruits. The fruit portion of a smoothie gives you pretty much everything that the whole fruit would have given you. The fiber content, for instance, is still intact.

Whole fruit, by the way, is basically the same now as it was 20,000 years ago, prior to the adoption of agricultural practices. Planting and cultivating fruit orchards have done nothing to change the nutrient profiles of fruits, and so our bodies are perfectly adapted to eat them.

CIGARETTES AND ALCOHOL

One of our favorite songs by the now defunct rock band Oasis is "Cigarettes and Alcohol." However, you may rest assured that cigarettes and alcohol were not on the "playlist" of our Paleo ancestors who went their whole lives without ever seeing a single tobacco product or alcoholic beverage. For modern day humans, cigarettes and alcohol present serious health risks. In fact, not only do cigarettes and alcohol put your arteries and internal organs at risk, they may undermine your attempts to lose weight or to even maintain your current weight.

In the case of cigarettes, while they may act in some cases as an appetite suppressant, they have been found to cause abdominal fat formation. As we have learned, the type of abdominal fat known as visceral fat may present a number of significant health risks, including heart disease, diabetes, stroke and even some forms of cancer. Also, nobody seeks out an increase in belly fat for cosmetic reasons, and we doubt that you have any desire to increase your waist size. Therefore, we recommend that you steer clear of tobacco products.

It is important for us to point out that, in addition to increasing belly fat, cigarettes have been found to increase the likelihood of developing several kinds of cancers, particularly lung cancer. In fact, smoking causes an estimated 90% of all lung cancer deaths in men and 80% of all lung cancer deaths in women.

In addition to causing cancer, smoking has been found to increase the risk of coronary heart disease by 2-to-4 times, the risk of stroke by 2-to-4 times and the risk of dying from chronic obstructive lung diseases (such as chronic bronchitis and emphysema) by 12-to-13 times. Even if you were not trying to lose weight, cigarettes represent a nightmare for your health.

Alcohol is not exactly a beauty queen when it comes to your health and losing weight. In the final analysis, alcohol offers little more than empty calories. While the antioxidants found in red wine may offer some nutritional value, you are better off getting your antioxidants by drinking pomegranate juice or by eating blueberries.

There are other health risks associated with the consumption of alcohol. Alcohol has also been found to cause damage to both the brain (especially in women) and the liver. While being touted for aiding in heart health at moderate intake levels, alcohol can even damage cardiovascular system at significant consumption levels. Finally, the National Cancer Institute points to alcohol as a risk factor for cancers of the mouth, esophagus, pharynx, larynx, liver and breast. So, do yourself a favor and avoid alcohol whenever possible.

THE RAW FOOD MYTH

Some people incorrectly assume that, 20,000 years ago, our ancestors were eating nothing but raw food. This leads them to think that our bodies are better adapted to eat raw food rather than cooked food. It turns out, however, that while our ancestors did not have agriculture 20,000 years ago, they had no shortage of fire, and they used it to cook their food. As a result, our bodies adapted to eat cooked rather than raw food. In fact, our bodies actually do a better job of assimilating food that is cooked rather than served raw, and cooked food may have accelerated our evolution as a species.

The nutrients in the food we eat tend to be more bioavailable to us when that food is cooked rather than eaten raw. Bioavailability refers to the percentage of a nutrient that is capable of being absorbed by tissues in the body and made available for use or storage. This simply means that, in general, when you eat raw food, your body is not getting the most out of it. Interestingly, both boiling and steaming preserve antioxidants better than frying, but boiling is better than all of the other methods of cooking—though just slightly better than steaming. Boiling, it turns out, reigns supreme.

HELPFUL HINT

There is one possible exception to this rule. It appears that broccoli should be eaten raw or *al dente* in order to receive all of its cancer-fighting effects, perhaps because cooking tends to diminish the Vitamin C content of food. More research is needed to confirm that this is the case.

WE KNOW WHAT YOU MIGHT BE THINKING

Are you asking the question, "What about yogurt?" The production of yogurt, after all, required the invention of agriculture. In order to make yogurt, people had to herd dairy-producing animals, milk them, apply live cultures to that milk and then wait. Yogurt was nowhere to be seen 20,000 years ago, long before domesticated livestock was first milked.

Despite the relative modernity of yogurt, however, the proteins and carbohydrates in milk have always served as the perfect food source for baby mammals. Moreover, scientists have recently determined that an adaptation in human evolution occurred approximately 10,000 years ago somewhere near modern-day Turkey. It was an adaptation that allowed humans to tolerate lactose throughout their lives, and not only in infancy. It is an adaptation known as lactase persistence. Thus, yogurt has its basis in a food source—milk—that we are perfectly evolved to eat. In fact, yogurt is even easier to digest than milk because the biological process used to make yogurt breaks down most of the lactose. We may, therefore, forgive yogurt for being a somewhat modern invention. It fits nicely into the Paleo Menu.

CHAPTER 4

GENIUS FOODS

"Genius Foods" are essentially normal foods that, from a nutritional standpoint, have one or more stellar qualities. Also, eating Genius Foods will make it easy for you to reach your nutritional goals. For weight-loss purposes, yogurt is the brightest star in the Genius Foods constellation, but we should not ignore other Genius Foods. Below, you will find just a few examples of Genius Foods. There are many others that are not listed here. The importance of Genius Foods is that their nutrient density gives us more nutrient bang for our calorie buck when we eat them. If you are going to put something into your mouth, consider making it a Genius Food.

ALMONDS

Almonds are loaded with one of the good fats—monounsaturated fat. They are also loaded with fiber (4 grams of fiber per cup). Your body needs dietary fat in order to be healthy, and consuming monounsaturated fat is especially good for your body.

APPLES

Apples contain pectin, which is a soluble fiber that can lower total cholesterol by as much as 10% and raise good cholesterol by as much as 10%. In addition to improving your cholesterol levels, apples contain flavonoids that have both antioxidant and anti-inflammatory properties.

AVOCADOS

Avocados come to us from central America by way of the Aztecs. They are a type of fruit that is rich in potassium, folic acid, magnesium and vitamin E. Avocados have also earned the right to boast of their high fiber content. Fiber improves our lipid profile and helps us to feel full.

Avocados are also loaded with good fat, namely, monounsaturated fat. In fact, not only are they loaded with monounsaturated fat, they are loaded with one of the best types of monounsaturated fat, oleic acid, which is also found in extra-virgin olive oil. Oleic acid appears to improve a person's lipid profile. A study found that after one week, a group on a diet that featured avocados enjoyed a drop in both total and LDL cholesterol (the bad kinds of cholesterol that cause hardening of the arteries) when compared to those in the control group that were not eating avocados. Significantly, there was also an 11% boost in HDL cholesterol in the experimental group. HDL cholesterol is the beneficial kind of cholesterol that reverses hardening of the arteries. So, follow the recipe for Mexicali Avocado Dip with Greek Yogurt in Section 5, and put a little into the next Mexican dish you eat. It truly is good for what ails you.

BEANS

If you are looking for a good source of protein that will not harm your cardiovascular health or cause cancer, you will be hard pressed to do better than you can with beans. Among other advantages over other sources of protein, beans have high levels of fiber. They also contain B vitamins, such as folic acid. In addition, they contain the phytonutrients that you can only get from consuming vegetables. Finally, they have very low glycemic indexes, such as garbanzo beans (also known as chickpeas), that have the extremely low glycemic index of 10.

A study in *Journal of the American College of Nutrition* found that people consuming 3/4 of one cup of beans per day have lower blood pressure and smaller waist sizes than those who skip beans in favor of other proteins. If you are trying to lose belly fat and weight around the midsection, then you should definitely be eating beans.

The domesticated garbanzo has the highest amount of the amino acid arginine of all foods. Arginine is the source our bodies use for nitric oxide synthesis, and this is one of the reasons that the Greek Yogurt Diet gives superb cardiovascular health. Arginine will soften and dilate our blood vessels and cause mitochondria to proliferate in our muscle cells. Both of these features make arginine very popular with body builders.

BLUEBERRIES

Blueberries have the ability to lower cholesterol but that is just the beginning. Blueberries are jam packed with antioxidants and flavonoids. The flavonoids present in blueberries happen to be so powerful that they can actually prevent cancer. In addition, blueberries are scientifically proven to improve memory. Most importantly, at least for the purposes of this book, berries in general contain plant chemicals called anthocyanins (pronounced ann-tho-SIGH-a-nins) that may suppress the formation of abdominal fat. If you are trying to maintain weight loss, then berries are your allies.

BLOOD ORANGES

Traditionally, blood oranges are grown in the foothills of Mount Etna in Sicily. The characteristic red pigment in blood oranges has been associated with improved cardiovascular health, controlling diabetes and reducing obesity. The pigments are anthocyanins, chemicals that colour red, purple and blue fruits. Thus, blood oranges possess qualities similar to blueberries.

In a 2010 study, blood orange juice helped animal subjects stave off obesity. While on a high-fat diet, the subjects developed 30% less white fat than animals given water or ordinary orange juice. Another study, conducted at the Catholic University of the Sacred Heart in Campobasso, Italy, found that people eating a high-fat breakfast accompanied with two cups of blood orange juice were less at risk from blood clotting three hours later. Arterial stiffness and levels of harmful triglyceride blood fats were also minimized as a result of drinking blood orange juice. Of course, we recommend eating whole oranges over drinking orange juice.

BROCCOLI

Broccoli is loaded with organic compounds that can have a positive impact on our health. Broccoli has been proven in preliminary studies to prevent tumors from forming and even to shrink tumors that have already formed. To get the full anti-cancer effects, it may be best to eat broccoli uncooked or slightly cooked (*al dente*). On top of its ability to fight cancer, broccoli enjoys the low glycemic index of just 15. It is low in calories yet high in fiber. Broccoli is a Genius Food if ever there was one.

CINNAMON

Cinnamon is a spice harvested from the inner bark of certain trees found on the island of Sri Lanka. The spice has been shown to improve the blood glucose levels and lipid profiles of people with type 2 diabetes, according to the National Institute of Health. Also, cinnamon has been proven to have powerful anti-viral effects. Finally, cinnamon shows some very initial promise at slowing the progression of Alzheimer's disease.

Be careful, though. Too much cinnamon may damage the liver. Fortunately, researchers at Tel Aviv University have developed a method of extracting the beneficial portion of cinnamon and separating it from the toxic substance (called cinnamaldehyde) found in it. While it may eventually be possible to purchase cinnamon that has been refined in this manner for health purposes, you may need to limit your cinnamon intake in the meantime.

CURCUMIN

Curcumin is found in turmeric spice, which is a member of the ginger family. Turmeric may be harvested in the forests of South and Southeast Asia. Turmeric plays a pivotal role in a variety of Thai and Indian dishes as it serves as the chief ingredient in almost every kind of curry. Despite the fact that it is a component of a common spice, curcumin appears to have powerful medicinal qualities that are anything but common.

One of curcumin's major health benefits appears to be that it appears to fight cancers, specifically the growth of tumors. It may also work to reduce kidney inflammation. In addition, it may be effective as a treatment for type 2 diabetes. Finally, it is now known to stimulate our brain's neurotrophic growth factors, which are responsible for the growth and survival of developing neurons and for the maintenance of mature neurons.

EGGPLANTS

Eggplant comes to our plates loaded with fiber as well as a full array of B vitamins. The antioxidants contained in purple are not only strong enough to turn the vegetable's skin purple, they may also be protective of our brain cells and help to keep our lipids (blood fats and cholesterol) at healthy levels.

EXTRA VIRGIN OLIVE OIL

Extra virgin olive oil contains the most health-promoting type of monounsaturated fat, oleic acid, making extra virgin olive oil the most healthful of all vegetable oils. It is also loaded with Vitamin E, antioxidants, and an anti-inflammatory agent called oleocanthal (pronounced oh-lee-oh-CAN-thel). Extra virgin olive oil has the ability to simultaneously cause a drop in bad cholesterol and prevent oxidation of the bad cholesterol that remains. It may also play a role in preventing certain types of cancer.

Not only are oleic acid and oleocanthal good for you, new research suggests that the smell alone of extra virgin olive oil can help you to lose weight. Merely the fragrance of olive oil, which contains aroma compounds such as hexanal, was found to trigger brain chemicals that help us feel full. People in a study that consumed olive-oil flavored yogurt ate less of other foods and also displayed better responses to glucose tolerance tests than the people consuming unflavored yogurt. In light of the fact that blood sugar is part of what controls hunger and satiation, extra virgin olive oil can be profoundly helpful for weight loss purposes. In addition, a study in *Obesity* showed that eating olive oil increased levels of a hormone in the body that breaks down body fat.

Be careful, though. Lower grades of olive oil are routinely mislabeled as extra virgin in order to fetch a higher price from consumers. This means that, once again, you need to do your homework on brands before bringing a product home to your kitchen.

FISH OIL

Fish oil is important due to the health benefits of the long-chain Omega-3s that it contains. For one thing, Omega-3s play a key role in the construction of cell membranes. Consider the fact that cell membranes are 95% fat. If the body lacked fatty acids, then the body would not have cells. Also, Omega-3s keep the heart working by acting on the signaling membranes in cardiac cells. In addition, Omega-3s affect how cells interact with each other. Omega-3s can even have an impact on how genes function.

There may be an even more exciting reason to consume fish oil, namely, weight loss. Researchers in Australia reviewed studies looking at the ability of long-chain Omega-3s to help us lose weight. They found evidence of improvements in blood circulation that they speculated that long-chain Omega-3s might aid in the delivery of nutrients to skeletal muscle tissue, which is largely responsible for burning the body's stores of fat. In addition, they noted enhanced fat oxidation and energy expenditure and, at the same time, reduced fat deposition. A reduction in fat deposition means that it was harder for the subjects to gain weight, and so long-chain Omega-3s may play a big role in helping you to maintain your weight loss once you have achieved it. Intriguingly, the researchers also found evidence of changes in gene expression that shifted the metabolism toward increased natural growth of lean tissue.

You may obtain fish oil by eating salmon, halibut and tuna, as well as by consuming other forms of aquatic life to varying degrees. You may also consider supplementing your dietary fish oil with molecularly distilled cod liver oil. We recommend consuming one tablespoonful per day of fish oil in one form or another.

> ## IMPORTANT HEALTH ALERT
>
> A study published in the *Journal of the National Cancer Institute* indicated that the consumption of fish oil may result in a greater risk of prostate cancer. Men, especially those who possess a family history of prostate cancer, should ask their physicians whether fish oil is safe for them.

GARLIC

When garlic is smashed, toothed or sliced, a powerful chemical known as allicin becomes active in it. Among other things, it appears that allicin may reduce hardening of the arteries and fat deposition. In addition to allicin, garlic is loaded with other chemical agents—such as saponins and arginine—that have powerful health-promoting effects.

It has been proven that garlic reduces the clumping of platelets in the blood, lowers blood pressure and lowers levels of fat and bad cholesterol in the blood while possibly increasing good cholesterol. Putting it all together, these effects should reduce the chance of hardening of the arteries, heart attacks and stroke. On top of its cardiovascular benefits, garlic appears to lower the risk of getting cancer. Garlic is certainly fantastic for your health.

HONEY

While honey is full of sugar, it has additional nutrients that may be advantageous to our health thanks to the bees that manufacture it. When you need a sweetener for a recipe or in your tea, you should definitely consider using honey. In one study, athletes that used honey as a sweetener kept their blood sugar at better levels for two hours than athletes that used sugar. In addition, honey may raise levels of good cholesterol (HDL) while simultaneously lowering levels of harmful triglyceride blood fats and bad cholesterol (LDL). Honey may also help to keep the level of antioxidants in our blood riding high. Finally, honey contains a type of good sugars called oligosaccharides (pronounced ah-lee-go-SACK-uh-rides) similar to the FOS found in yogurt that may contribute to having a healthful balance of bacteria and other microbes in the digestive system. When you are choosing a honey, seek out one that is darker in color. It will tend to promote health better than lighter colored honey.

KALE

Kale is a cruciferous vegetable and is considered to be similar to a type of wild cabbage. It is full of fiber and antioxidants. It also has a high level of Vitamin K. Like other cruciferous vegetables, kale is a source of a chemical that aids in the DNA repair of cells and appears to block the growth of cancer cells. Kale is definitely a vegetable that a genius would eat.

KIWIFRUIT

Kiwifruit contains impressive amounts of Vitamin B-3, Vitamin C, Vitamin E and powerful, plant-based antioxidants like flavonoids. Kiwis also serve as storehouses for chlorophyll, glutathione, pectin, potassium and fiber. You could do a lot worse nutritionally, especially when you consider the fact that the kiwifruit is one of the most nutrient-dense foods on the planet, giving you lots of nutrient bang for your calorie buck.

POMEGRANATES

Pomegranates are chock full of flavonoids, Vitamin C, Vitamin B-6 and potassium. In addition, the juice of the pomegranate might contain 2-to-3 times the antioxidant potency of green tea. It has even been found to aid the cardiovascular system by limiting the oxidation of LDL cholesterol. Even more amazingly, preliminary research indicates that pomegranates may reverse hardening of the arteries.

PUMPKINS

Pumpkins are vegetables that manage to be low in calories yet high in fiber and carotenoids (such as beta carotene). In fact, the orange color of pumpkins tips us off to their high carotenoid content. Carotenoids are fat-soluble chemical compounds that decrease your risk for heart disease as well as reduce your risk for a various kinds of cancer. You will be giving yourself a treat and not a trick if you pretend that it is October every month and eat pumpkins all-year round.

SPINACH

Spinach contains antioxidants, coenzyme-Q10, multiple types of Vitamin B, minerals, chlorophyll and short-chain Omega-3s. Scientists have discovered that the more spinach people eat, the less chance they have of getting many types of cancer. Also, all of the antioxidants present in spinach work in concert to fight against hardening of the arteries and other diseases of the cardiovascular system.

STEEL-CUT OATMEAL

Old-fashioned, steel-cut oatmeal comes from whole grain groats (the inner portion of the oat kernel) that have been cut into pieces. Because the groats have been cut rather than flattened (as they are in instant oatmeal), the oats require more time to be digested, and that gives us a feeling of fullness that lasts an extra amount of time. As you may have guessed, this is all due to fiber content. A single serving of steel-cut oatmeal supplies you with 4-to-5 grams of fiber.

Steel-cut oatmeal is superior to instant oatmeal in part due to its glycemic index. It boasts a glycemic index of 42, whereas instant oatmeal has the relatively high glycemic index of 65.

Perhaps most importantly, steel-cut oatmeal helps to eliminate fat and cholesterol from the body. Studies show that for people with high cholesterol levels, consuming just 3 grams of soluble oat fiber per day typically lowers their total cholesterol numbers by 8-to-23%.

One benefit of eating a whole grain like steel-cut oatmeal is that it can reduce belly fat. A study published in *The American Journal of Clinical Nutrition* in 2008 showed that a restricted calorie diet rich in whole grains had a powerful effect on the fat deposited around the middle of the body. The subjects that ate whole grains but no processed grains, in addition to five servings of fruits and vegetables, three servings of low-fat dairy, and two servings of lean meat, fish, or poultry, lost more weight from the abdominal area than the control group that ate the same diet, but also ate highly processed grains instead of whole grains.

TEA

As we have learned, black tea has been proven to help lower cortisol levels, and that is reason enough to drink it. But there are many other reasons to drink tea. Tea has been proven to improve the health of our hearts, drop our chances for strokes and decrease our blood pressure. It can also reduce our chances of getting cancer. Tea may even keep osteoporosis at bay. In addition, green tea may stimulate the fat-burning, brown fat cells. Finally, the effects of tea may also have an effect on the skin. It turns out that tea may actually reduce damage of the skin caused by rays from the sun. This would translate into fewer wrinkles and fewer incidents of skin cancer.

Keep in mind that there are basically two types of tea that you can drink for health benefits: green tea, which comes from unfermented leaves, and black tea, which comes from fermented leaves. The fermentation process is responsible for creating two different sets of antioxidants.

For a while, people believed that green tea was more beneficial than black tea. This was partly due to the fact that a specific antioxidant, epigallocatechin gallate (EGCG), exists in greater amounts in green tea than it does in black tea. Also, certain kinds of antioxidants undergo chemical changes as a byproduct of the fermentation process. This made many suspect that the flavonoids in black tea might be inactive.

Despite all of the concerns over black tea, however, studies have shown that its flavonoids are extremely bioactive and yield many health benefits. Instead of EGCG, black tea is loaded with health-promoting theaflavins and thearubigens that get created during the fermentation of the leaves. As we have also discussed, black tea can help reduce cortisol levels.

There may be an additional reason to drink black tea. Black tea contains chlorogenic acids, and initial studies indicate that chlorogenic acids (CGAs) may promote weight loss. In addition to making an appearance in black tea, CGAs may also be found in green coffee beans, lowbush blueberries, sunflower seeds and potato skins, to varying degrees.

CGAs appear to help us to lose weight in three ways. First, they seem to delay the entry of glucose (sugar) into the bloodstream. Second, they may stimulate the efforts of the body's own fat-burning enzymes. Third, CGAs appear to minimize the amount of lipids (fats) in the body.

By delaying the release of glucose into the bloodstream, CGAs essentially lower the glycemic index of whatever food you are eating. CGAs also have the effect of inhibiting the enzymes that break down carbohydrates into sugar. If you are being careful to eat foods with a lower glycemic index, CGAs may launch those efforts into hyperdrive.

In addition to slowing the entry of sugar into the bloodstream, CGAs reduce the fat and cholesterol in your body. In one study conducted in Beijing, the levels of fasting serum triglyceride, free fatty acids, total cholesterol and low density lipoprotein cholesterol were significantly lower in the subjects receiving CGAs.

Not only do CGAs reduce the amount of fat and cholesterol in your body, CGAs appear to switch on the body's own fat-burning enzymes. This improves your body's ability to burn fat.

At the same time that your fat-burning enzymes are switched on, CGAs switch off the body's fat-making enzymes. So, it appears that your body stops stockpiling fat, and simultaneously starts burning fat in response to the consumption of CGAs.

In a study published in the *Journal of International Medical Research*, subjects given instant coffee enriched with CGAs may have demonstrated the effects of CGAs. First, their absorption of glucose decreased by 6.9% compared with the control group. Those drinking normal or decaffeinated instant coffee did not enjoy the same reduction in glucose absorption.

A second study performed by the same investigators looked at the effect of CGAs on the body mass of 30 overweight people. Those taking CGAs lost nearly 12 pounds on average while those not receiving CGAs lost only 3.7 pounds on average. So, consuming CGAs—without making any changes to diet or exercise—can cause modest weight loss.

We, therefore, recommend that you drink both types of tea. Drink black tea up to thirty minutes before each meal and then drink green tea at other times throughout the day. That way you maximize the health benefits of each and get a wide range of flavonoids.

While caffeine is generally something that you want to avoid, steer clear of decaffeinated teas. Unfortunately, the decaffeination process destroys much of the flavonoid content of tea. To avoid the problems associated with excessive caffeine intake, regulate the amount of tea that you drink throughout the day so that you do not accidentally consume too much caffeine. This is especially important when bedtime nears. The good news is that tea contains much less caffeine than coffee.

TOMATOES

Tomatoes contain Vitamin A, Vitamin C and Vitamin K. Tomatoes may also boast of high levels of the antioxidant lycopene, which gives tomatoes their red color. To get the full benefits of lycopene, cook your tomatoes at high heat and then add a little bit of fat—preferably in the form of extra virgin olive oil—before eating them.

WALNUTS

Of all the nuts, walnuts contain the greatest levels of antioxidants. Also, walnuts have high levels of the medium-chain,

Omega-3 fat called alpha-linolenic acid. Alpha-linolenic acid is extremely beneficial to our cardiovascular systems as the body turns it into a long-chain Omega-3 fat called EPA. Finally, eating any kind of nut has been shown by Harvard scientists to lower our risk for developing type 2 diabetes. In fact, eating a handful of nuts five times per week lowered the risk for type 2 diabetes by nearly 30%.

WESTERN YELLOW ONIONS

All onions are loaded with antioxidants, and onions come in many varieties. Of the many types of onions that exist, western yellow onions have the most antioxidants—more than 10 times the amount of flavonoids found in western white onions, for example. All of that antioxidant power pays off big. For one thing, it appears that onions can lower our chance of coronary heart disease by up to 20%. In addition, it appears that they can help to fight off cancer of the brain, colon, esophagus, lung and stomach. Due to their anti-inflammatory effects, onions can be used to help treat asthma and both types of arthritis.

YOGURT

Last, but certainly not least, yogurt is the most ingenious of the Genius Foods for weight loss and weight maintenance purposes. It is high in protein, low in sugar and low in carbohydrates. It is also available in a fat-free variety. Most importantly, whey protein accounts for much of the protein found in yogurt that is produced properly. Whey protein reduces the level of the stress hormone called cortisol in our bodies, allowing us to lose weight faster—especially belly fat—while maintaining more bone density and lean body mass than dieting alone. It is also full of FOS that, like the oligosaccharides found in honey, may be responsible for improving the healthful balance between bacteria and other microbes in the gut.

CHAPTER 5

DRINK AND EAT TO CONTROL CORTISOL

There are four substances that we can consume that may reduce the amount of the stress hormone called cortisol found in our bodies. The first substance that reduces the amount of cortisol in our bodies is black tea. A second substance is fish oil (specifically, the long-chain Omega-3s contained in fish oil). A third substance is, of all things, dark chocolate. Fourth, yogurt works to control cortisol levels.

BLACK TEA

A study conducted at the University College of London and published in the September 2006 issue of *Psychopharmacology* looked at the ability of tea to relieve stress. Healthy male subjects in the test group drank 4 cups of black tea versus those in the control group that drank a placebo. Prior to drinking black tea—and during the treatments—all of the experimental subjects took stress tests. The researchers reported that the men drinking black tea had lower levels of the stress hormone called cortisol after performing stressful tasks compared with the men in the control group.

In addition to affecting cortisol levels, black tea reduces the amount of cholesterol in your body. It may also have a powerful effect on the way that your body processes the food that you eat.

In light of black tea's apparent ability to promote weight loss, we recommend that you drink black tea up to thirty minutes before each meal. Then, drink *green* tea at other times of the day in order to obtain the many benefits of drinking both types tea.

Keep in mind that you will want to reduce your overall tea intake as your bedtime nears because any caffeine in your tea could make it difficult to sleep. Unfortunately, decaffeinated tea is not an acceptable substitute for caffeinated tea due to the fact that the decaffeination process destroys much of the flavonoid content of tea. However, you do not need to be overly concerned about the caffeine content of tea because its caffeine levels are relatively minimal.

OMEGA-3S

In the June 2003 issue of *Diabetes Metabolism,* research conducted in France looked at the effects of the long-chain, Omega-3s found in fish oil on stress hormones brought on by psychological stressors. The researchers observed that participants taking 7.2 grams of fish oil per day for three weeks had lower cortisol levels after undergoing a stress test than the subjects taking a placebo.

We recommend consuming Omega-3s on a daily basis by taking molecularly distilled supplements to ensure that you get adequate levels. You can also obtain Omega-3s by eating wild salmon. Farmed salmon does not contain the same high levels of Omega-3s found in wild salmon, but it still has more Omega-3s than other kinds of fish, including tuna, cod, bass and tilapia. It is typically referred to simply as Atlantic salmon because that is the variety that is being farmed in pens. No wild salmon comes directly from the Atlantic these days because wild salmon in the Atlantic Ocean is now protected from harvesting. The varieties of wild salmon from the Pacific that you will see in markets and restaurants are called chinook (or, king), sockeye, coho (or, silver) and chum (or, pink). For sustainable ecological purposes, line-caught salmon is the best that you can buy.

In addition to salmon, Omega-3s can be found in abundance in halibut, tuna, flax, walnuts and soybeans. It should be noted that consuming flax, walnuts and soybeans will only give you short-chain Omega-3s, but your body has the ability to convert some short-chain Omega-3s into long-chain Omega-3s (though probably not enough for our purposes and so you will likely need to supplement with other sources).

HELPFUL HINT

It is more cost effective to purchase molecularly distilled cod liver oil in liquid form than it is to purchase capsules or to eat salmon daily. My recommended daily dose of molecularly distilled cod liver oil is approximately 1 tablespoon. In comparison with capsules, you would need to take fifteen one-gram capsules just to get the equivalent of a single tablespoon. The advantage of molecular distillation is that it both purifies and removes odor in order to improve taste. A brand that we recommend is Nordic Naturals. We feel comfortable recommending Nordic Naturals because we personally know the company located in Watsonville, California. They purchase far-north, North Sea cod liver oil and purify the oil by molecular distillation (CO_2 distillation). We know the caliber of their products, and we also know that, in most cases, you can find their products at a natural foods market near you.

DARK CHOCOLATE

Consuming dark chocolate, in small doses, might reduce cortisol levels. Scientists at the Nestle Research Center in Germany presented a study in the October 2009 issue of the *Journal of Proteome Research* reported that people ingesting 1.4 ounces of dark chocolate per day for two weeks showed decreases in cortisol levels.

In addition to dark chocolate's ability to affect cortisol levels, the flavonoid content in dark chocolate may have a number of additional health benefits. For instance, eating just 1-to-2 ounces of dark chocolate per day may actually lower both blood pressure and cholesterol levels. The antioxidants in chocolate may also protect the skin from ultraviolet rays and reduce the risk of experiencing dementia or stroke.

While we want you to avoid candy in general, dark chocolate, in moderation, has a number of virtues as we have already discussed. Limit your intake of dark chocolate to 1-to-2 ounces per day, which would be an amount that is about the size of your thumb tip. Otherwise, you will discover that too much dark chocolate is too much of a good thing, making it difficult to lose weight. For one thing, dark chocolate is high in fat. Dark chocolate tends to also be high in sugar. Due to its sugar content, we recommend eating your daily dark chocolate at the end of your largest meal of the day in order to minimize the effects of its relatively high glycemic index. Choose non-oxidized chocolate products that preserve beneficial flavonoids. Alkalai-processed chocolate has great flavor but no flavonoids.

Both Mars and Hershey manufacture some of their chocolates in a way that preserves these flavonoids, and those products may sometimes be identified by their special labeling. In the case of Mars chocolate products (such as Dove), look for a reference on the label to Mars' proprietary COCOAPRO® process or the words "Natural Source of Cocoa Flavanols." In the case of Hershey's, choose its Extra Dark chocolate bar or its Special Dark Cocoa. Other than Mars and Hershey products, we would favor boutique manufacturers that employ fresh processing rather than alkali processing. Dutch-processed cocoa, for instance, requires the use of alkali processing and should be avoided.

YOGURT

It turns out that the whey protein that may be present in yogurt is high in alpha-lactalbumin. Alpha-lactalbumin is a type of whey protein that acts directly on cortisol levels. In a study published in the *American Journal of Clinical Nutrition*, researchers from the TNO Nutrition and Food Research Institute in the Netherlands examined the impact of alpha-lactalbumin on cortisol levels under stress by looking at vulnerable subjects. Researchers found that people consuming a diet rich in alpha-lactalbumin enjoyed reductions in cortisol levels after undergoing a short period of stress in contrast to people consuming a diet high in casein protein (another protein found in milk) who did not enjoy reductions in cortisol levels.

CHAPTER 6

SNACK LIKE A GENIUS

It is probably worth mentioning, more than once even, that all snacking should be done in moderation. In fact, you should try to limit yourself to no more than two snacks a day, with each snack containing between 100 and 200 calories, depending upon the amount of calories that you are consuming in your meals. Having said that, all of these snacking options, with the exception of snacks with a high sugar or fat content, are fairly harmless. This is especially true when it comes to snacking on fruits and vegetables with low glycemic indexes. So, by all means, munch away on some cherries.

KALE CHIPS

Kale chips have the thinness and crunch of potato chips, but they are much better for your health. One cup of kale chips should contain fewer than 100 calories (see the recipe for making your own kale chips in Section 6).

HUMMUS

Hummus, made from garbanzo beans (or, chickpeas) and, ideally, extra virgin olive oil (which is loaded with oleic acid—the best type of monounsaturated fat), makes for the perfect snack food. As we have learned, hummus has the unbelievably low glycemic index of 6. Dip carrots, broccoli and cauliflower into it. Or, try chips made from beans, like Beanitos®, which are high in fiber and protein and simultaneously low in fat and sodium. Choose Pinto Bean & Flax Beanitos® as they are high in Omega-3s. Like everything else, hummus needs to be eaten in moderation. One quarter of a cup of hummus (see the recipe in Section 6) and some veggies or Beanitos® to dip into it should contain fewer than 100 calories.

VEGGIES AND DIP

Eat one cup of fresh vegetables with 1 tablespoon of Goddess Dip (see the recipe in Section 5).

OLIVES

Olives are high in oleocanthal, which is a substance that has the ability to simultaneously cause a drop in bad cholesterol and prevent oxidation of the bad cholesterol that remains. It may also play a role in preventing certain types of cancer. Ten olives of any kind should contain fewer than 100 calories.

TURKEY BREAST LETTUCE WRAP

Have some skinless, free-range turkey breast with hummus and/or Greek Yogurt "Mayonnaise" (see the recipe in Section 5) wrapped in lettuce.

EDAMAME

One-half cup of unshelled edamame should have no more than 130 calories. Edamame are young, green soy beans. Look for them in your frozen food aisle.

PEANUTS

Have a one-ounce serving of peanuts. The peanut, which is a member of the legume family, has bragging rights to the extremely low glycemic index of 7. In addition to its low glycemic index, the peanut is a good source of vitamin E, fiber, magnesium and folic acid. It also serves as an excellent source of Vitamin B-3. Plus, one serving of peanuts contains 7 grams of protein. This nutrient profile makes peanuts an excellent snack food. The same is true for peanut butter. The next time you feel the need for a snack, have some peanuts or dip some celery or other vegetable into some peanut butter. If you must eat your peanut butter with bread, then spread some peanut butter onto a single slice of multi-grain bread. On a side note, always make sure that your peanut butter has a low sugar content. Commercially made peanut butter can be a hidden source of sugar.

CINNAMON RICOTTA CHEESE WITH APPLES

Mix some cinnamon powder and some sweetener to taste into a one-quarter cup of fat-free ricotta cheese. Then, add half an apple cut into slices and enjoy a sweet little snack. Ricotta contains whey protein because it is, in fact, made from whey. However, ricotta does not contain the same high levels of whey protein found in yogurt.

YOGURT ICE POPS

Yogurt ice pops can help us to reach the goals outlined in this book due to their whey protein content. The only downside to them is their possible sugar content. Taken in moderation, however, they are an acceptable snack food for the Greek Yogurt Diet (see the recipe for making your own yogurt ice pops in Section 5).

GENIUS FOODS

Try snacking on some blueberries or popping the contents of a one-ounce package of almonds into your mouth. These and other kinds of Genius Foods are jam-packed with health-promoting substances. Therefore, all Genius Foods make for the perfect snack when eaten in moderation.

Genius Foods and other snacks become even better if you are able to mix them with Greek yogurt. Keep in mind that plain Greek yogurt may be used to create either a savory snack or a sweet snack. It is all a matter of preparation, and the only limit is your imagination. If you are looking for ideas, stop by the Chobani SoHo store on Prince Street in Manhattan. There you may find everything from peanut butter and jelly in Greek yogurt to smoked salmon and dill mixed into Greek yogurt.

CHAPTER 7

PORTION CONTROL MADE EASY

Portion control means that you start limiting the amount that you eat based on recommended portion sizes. Without imposing controls on the size of the portions that we eat, we might be unintentionally "super-sizing" our portions, and eating far more than we should. Our aim is to eat smaller portions of everything that we eat.

There are some strategies that we all can use to help us with portion control. One strategy is to plan meals in advance. Some would go so far as to recommend that once you have mapped out a proper meal with properly sized portions you should eat the same meals or the same portions of components of meals week after week. For instance, you could eat two scrambled egg whites and an apple for breakfast every Monday for the rest of your life. It would be the same-sized apple and the same portion size of egg whites. This is a good strategy, but it might become a bit too monotonous for some eaters. See if you can make some version of this strategy work for you.

Another technique is to use smaller plates. Most dinner plates are about 13 inches in diameter. Try using a 9-inch plate, instead. If anyone asks, just tell them that the plates are for Spanish tapas, which they might well be depending upon what you are cooking that evening.

HELPFUL HINT

A study found that if the color of your plate matches the color of the food that you are serving, you tend to serve less food to yourself or others. The suspected reason is that by reducing the color contrast between your plate and your food, your brain is tricked into thinking that there is more food on the plate than there actually is. So, the next time you serve eggplant, for instance, serve it on a purple plate.

If you accidentally eat too large a portion from time to time, it will not be the end of your diet. You are in this for the long haul. Portion control is a lifestyle change that you should seek to adopt permanently. Do not let a temporary setback fluster you.

DRINK A COLD PINT
BEFORE EACH MEAL

Let's talk about water. Researchers at Virginia Tech published a study on the effects of drinking water on weight loss in *Obesity* in 2010. They found that drinking water before a meal had a powerful effect. One group of subjects drank slightly more than one pint of water shortly before each of three daily meals. The others were given no instructions on what to drink. Before the study, all subjects had been consuming between 1,800 and 2,200 calories a day. When the study started, researchers limited the total daily consumption of the women to 1,200 calories, while allowing the male subjects to consume 1,500. After three months the group that drank a little over a pint of water before meals had lost a little over 15 pounds each, on average, while those in the control group lost only 11 pounds. Please note that if you are drinking black tea or some other beverage before a meal, you may reduce the amount of water that you are drinking accordingly.

There is another reason to drink so much H_2O. Water consumption has been shown to increase metabolic rates. A study conducted at the Franz-Volhard Clinical Research Center in Berlin looked at the effect of drinking water on energy expenditures.

After drinking approximately 17 ounces of water, the subjects' metabolic rates increased by 30% for both men and women. This means that they were burning calories at an increased rate. The increases began within 10 minutes of water consumption and reached a maximum about 30 to 40 minutes after drinking the water.

The researchers calculated that a person that increases his or her water consumption by a little over a pint a day would burn an extra 17,400 calories per year for a weight loss of approximately five pounds on an annual basis. While the metabolic gains may not add up to a huge amount of calories, every small thing that you can do to lose weight helps. The scientists emphasized that up to 40% of the increase in calorie burning is caused by the body's attempt to heat the ingested water. This means that it is important to drink cold water rather than water at room temperature or warmer.

MEASURE YOUR FOOD WITH EVERYDAY OBJECTS

A good way to figure out portion sizes on the fly is to compare portions to familiar objects. By thinking of portions in those terms, the proper size becomes easy to visualize. Each item listed below is the equivalent of a single serving of that food. We will first look at vegetables, then grains, then dairy products, proteins, fruits, fats, sweets and finally mixed foods.

Vegetables. The correct portion size for baby carrots is one cup, but that might be hard to visualize. Instead of thinking about what a cup of baby carrots would look like, think of a tight cluster of baby carrots about the size and shape of a major league baseball (not a giant softball). That baseball-sized cluster roughly equals one portion. A cup of broccoli or a cup of leafy green vegetables should, likewise, each fit inside its own baseball to equal one portion. In the case of leafy green vegetables, they would be all scrunched up inside of a baseball. An ear of corn should be no longer than the length of a #2 pencil, or about 8 inches, which is equal to one portion size.

Grains. One cup of cooked pasta equals one portion size, and you may visualize it as the size of a major-league baseball. One-half cup of cooked rice or cooked couscous should fit inside of a standard-sized light bulb. A slice of whole grain bread should have dimensions no thicker, longer or wider than a cassette tape.

Dairy. The serving size of yogurt is one cup, which is equal to eight fluid ounces and should fill up a major league baseball. A half-cup of frozen yogurt or a half-cup of ice cream should each barely fit inside of a standard light bulb. Due to the saturated fat content of hard cheese, a single serving size is only 1.5 ounces, which should be no larger than a 9-volt battery or three standard-sized dice. That is one portion size of hard cheese.

Proteins. Three ounces of cooked, lean beef or three ounces of cooked chicken should each be no larger than a deck of playing cards. Three ounces of cooked fish should be no larger than a standard-sized checkbook, which is slightly larger than a deck of playing cards. One quarter of a cup of almonds, one quarter of a cup of walnuts or 2 tablespoons of hummus should each be about the size of a golf ball.

Fruits. One medium-sized apple is one portion and should be no larger than a tennis ball. You should be able to cram either a half cup of blueberries or a half cup of grapes into a light bulb. An ounce of any dried fruit should fit inside of a golf ball. One baseball should accommodate one cup of strawberries.

Fats. One tablespoon portion of butter, margarine, salad dressing or olives should be no larger than a ping-pong ball. Due to the saturated fat content of hard cheese, a single serving size is only 1.5 ounces, which should be no larger than a 9-volt battery or three standard-sized dice.

Sweets. A half cup of your favorite flavor of ice cream is one portion, and it should fit inside of a standard light bulb. A one-ounce portion of dark chocolate should be no bigger than a small package of dental floss. A cup of pudding equals one single serving, and it should fit neatly inside of a baseball.

Mixed Foods. The silhouette of one burrito should be no larger than the dimensions of a checkbook. One three-ounce hamburger should be no larger than a deck of playing cards. You should be able to pour one cup of chili or your favorite soup into a major league baseball. A single serving of French fries is 10 fries. Three ounces of meat loaf should be no larger than a deck of playing cards.

YOU HOLD THE ANSWER IN THE PALM OF YOUR HAND

Another simple way to exercise portion control over how much you eat is to use your own hand as a measurement tool. For instance, 3 ounces of lean beef or 3 ounces of cooked chicken should fit on one of your palms. One portion of pasta or one cup of popped popcorn should be no larger than the size of your fist. A tablespoon portion of peanut butter should be about the size of your thumb tip.

DINING OUT

When dining out, always remember to tell the host or waiter when you are seated that you do not want to be served any bread or rolls. An endless supply of highly processed bread is the last thing that you need when you are trying to lose weight. You might as well be eating sugar by the spoonful.

When attempting to use portion control, you obviously cannot control what size dishes restaurants decide to use. So, try to super-impose your memory of what your smaller-sized plate at home looks like onto the larger plate when you are dining out, and then eat smaller portions accordingly. Alternatively, order two nutritionally sound appetizers in place of an entree. Make sure that you avoid ordering appetizers that are little more than "fat bombs" (sorry, no deep-fried mozzarella sticks). Remind yourself that you are looking for two appetizers that contain vegetables, lean proteins, and health-promoting fats. Finally, always ask your waiter to bag up some portion of your meal to take with you. Avoid eating until the last bite. Later, you will have a nice snack to enjoy at home.

THE MYSTERY OF THE STARBUCKS® DIET

On September 13, 2013, NBC News' *today.com* reported that a librarian in Virginia named Christine Hall claimed to have lost 85 pounds by following what some are touting as the "Starbucks® Diet." Almost all of the food that she has eaten over the past couple of years has come from Starbucks®.

"A law librarian with two jobs, she gets her meals from the Starbucks right near work, where employees have cheered on the 5-foot, 4-inch Hall as she's gone from weighing 190 to a trim 114 pounds," reported *today.com*.

The factor that made the diet work for Ms. Hall is that she rigorously applied a very simple principle. The *today.com* report states that she "started keeping a written food diary and lost 10 pounds. By May 10, 2010, at 190 pounds, she discovered the MyPlate calorie tracker at livestrong.com and started buying all of her food from Starbucks."

Ms. Hall accomplished her goal by counting calories and using portion control which was made easy by the fact that Starbucks® gives everyone information on the exact number of calories and the nutrition facts of each of its menu items. Starbucks® was effective for Ms. Hall because she knew exactly how many calories she was getting with every order. She could add up what she was eating and make sure that she never over-ate.

Ms. Hall also made a concerted effort to make healthful choices, reserving treats like brownies for special occasions. She sought out menu items like the "Bistro Box" for lunch and opted for a panini as dinner. While not always ideal, her selections were not the worst choices she could have made, and marrying her food choices to a strict form of portion control allowed her to reach her weight-loss goals.

We can use Ms. Hall's example and be just as rigorous about controlling the amount of food that we put into our bodies. You should be able to obtain equally impressive results by simply counting calories and exercising portion control. Using an app to keep track of what you eat is also a good idea. There is much to learn from Ms. Hall's approach to losing weight, whether you are at Starbucks® or anywhere else.

HARA HACHI BU

Okinawa is one of the Ryukyu islands in Japan. The origins of the people first to arrive in Okinawa remains unknown. One theory is that they arrived from the Chinese mainland about 32,000 years ago, possibly crossing over on a land bridge that no longer exists. Over many centuries, there has also been an influx of people from the main island of Japan. Essentially, the genetics of the people of Okinawa is not much different from the genetics of people living in China and Japan. What makes them special is what they eat and how they live.

People eating the traditional diet of the island and following the traditional lifestyle of the island tend to live a very long time. In fact, they live an extraordinarily long time. Okinawa has about 34 centenarians (people that are 100 years of age or older) per 100,000 people. Compare that figure to the United States which only has about 17 centenarians per 100,000 people. The fact that Okinawa has twice as many centenarians as the United States represents a huge longevity gap between the two population groups. It tells us that we could be living a lot longer than we do.

Not only do people following the traditional Okinawan way of life enjoy longer lives than just about anyone anywhere else, they are much healthier. Okinawans are about 80% less likely to suffer from heart disease. They are 25% less likely to get breast or prostate cancer. In addition, they are 50% less likely to get colon cancer. They spend approximately 97% of their lives, on average, free of any disabilities whatsoever.

While there are many factors that help to explain why Okinawans live longer and healthier lives than most Americans, one factor is certainly diet. The traditional diet of Okinawa consists of green and yellow vegetables as 30% of total calories consumed. While the Japanese diet usually includes large quantities of rice, the Okinawans eat smaller amounts of rice, opting instead for sweet potato. The Okinawan diet reduces sugar by 75% and reduces grain consumption by 25% compared to the average Japanese dietary intake. Pork is highly valued but primarily eaten on holidays only. A typical meal in Okinawa would be based on plants rather than meat.

In addition to diet, there is one rule that Okinawans follow that is an elegantly simple form of portion control. It is so simple, in fact, that all of us can easily practice the rule, and it may result in all of us living longer and healthier lives. It is called the *Hara Hachi Bu* (pronounced HA-da HA-chee BOO) rule.

Hara Hachi Bu is the Okinawan way of saying, "Eat until you are 80% full." This is one of the simplest dietary rules that you are ever going to learn. The aspect that makes this rule so ingenious is that it compensates for the delay between the time that you eat and the time that your brain finally receives the message from the stomach that you are full. Because food travels so slowly to the stomach (it takes about 20 minutes), people tend to overeat because they simply do not realize that they have already eaten enough or, in many cases, more than enough. Their brain has simply not gotten the message, and so they still feel hungry.

The *Hara Hachi Bu* rule reduces the risk of overeating through the discipline of not trusting that last pang of hunger that you experience before you finish eating. When you feel 80% full, simply stop. Shortly thereafter, the message from your stomach will finally reach your brain and you will experience the feeling of satiety. By halting your eating at the 80% point and waiting for your brain to receive that message, you are now practicing the *Hara Hachi Bu* rule.

CHAPTER 8

EAT MINDFULLY TO LOSE WEIGHT FASTER

How many times have you sat down in front of the television set with a plate full of delicious food perched on your lap? Suddenly, your favorite show starts. You watch your program with rapt attention, taking in your favorite characters and not missing a word of dialogue. Your fork hits the plate and—somehow—all of your food is gone. You appear to have eaten it all without any memory of the food passing through your lips. While you know that you must have eaten what had been on your plate, you find that you are hungry again a short time later. In fact, you have a hard time convincing yourself that you did, in fact, eat at all. Sound familiar?

Practicing mindfulness immediately before, during and after you eat can have a profound impact on your eating habits. For one thing, it slows down the eating process. By slowing down, we give our food enough time to reach the stomach.

The stomach can then send signals to the brain that we have had enough to eat. It also helps us to remember that we have eaten later so that we can counteract impulses to eat with the thought: "But I've already eaten."

It also gives you a chance to contemplate exactly what it is that you are about to put into your mouth. When we give ourselves time to examine our food choices, we can exercise buyer's remorse. "Perhaps we do not need to be eating pizza right now," we might think just before taking our first bite, and decide to eat something more healthful instead. Or, even if we do not change our minds with the meal in front of us, taking time to think about what we are eating at the present meal will help us to make better food choices for future meals.

In fact, a small yet growing body of research has confirmed that taking the time to contemplate our food as we eat it will help us to lose pounds and choose better food options. Although food contemplation might sound like something reserved for a Zen retreat, science is starting to show us that being mindful when we eat can serve as a powerful aid for weight loss and healthful eating.

The idea is to turn off distractions like computers and television sets. Or, if you sometimes eat while driving (perhaps after picking up your food at a drive-through window), pull over to the side of the road. Wherever you are—and once it is safe to do so—slow your breathing down and begin to inhale a bit more deeply for about a minute or so just before eating. Close your eyes for a bit. Allow your mind to become calm and centered. Then, if you wish, open your eyes. Allow yourself to become aware of what you are about to eat: the smells, shapes and colors. Contemplate the work that people did in order to get your food's many ingredients into a grocery store and everything that went into its preparation. Become aware of the choices that you have made in what you are eating. Did you choose a healthful option? Are you about to eat food that is highly nutritious or are you about to fill up on empty calories?

When you take your first bite, become aware of the way it feels going into your mouth. Notice its temperature, feel and texture. Chew each bite slowly and thoroughly. Become aware of how each bite feels in your mouth. You want to create a memory. Focus on what you are doing as you eat. Allow yourself to fully enjoy what you are eating. Savor your food.

HELPFUL HINT

If you are still eating your food too quickly—even after practicing mindfulness—try setting an alarm or timer to go off twenty minutes after you take your first bite. Then, stretch out your meal and hold off on eating the last several bites until after the alarm sounds. You might find that you no longer have an appetite after the buzzer sounds, allowing you to forgo eating the remainder of your meal.

STAGE THE MEAL

Instead of cramming everything that you plan to eat onto a single plate, plate a single serving of one item of food on a small plate as your first course. Then, plate a second serving of that item or a single serving of another item of food on a small plate as your second course, and so forth. By serving yourself a multi-course meal, you are guaranteeing that you are paying more attention to what you are eating. You are also buying yourself more time for feelings of satisfaction to travel from your stomach to your brain so that you can stop eating earlier on in the meal.

USE FUN TRICKS TO CREATE MINDFULNESS

If you are right-handed, try eating with your left hand. If you are left-handed, try eating with your right hand. By placing your fork in your non-dominant hand, you can guarantee two things: You will need to slow down, and you will be forced to become more aware of the process.

Take yourself off of auto-pilot when you eat. Use a spoon or chopsticks when you would normally use a fork. Likewise, use a fork when you would normally use chopsticks. It will pull your mind into what you are doing and force you to become aware of what you are eating and exactly how much of it is going into your mouth. Studies show that these tricks result in significant decreases in calorie consumption.

THINK YOUR WAY THIN

Cognitive psychology is the study of mental processes such as attention, memory, perception and thinking. Studies from the field of cognitive psychology have shown that if you practice mindfulness while you eat in order to create memories and then later remind yourself of what you have eaten previously during the course of your day, then you will be more likely to eat less later than you otherwise would. Try to create a memory while you are eating. Then, before you eat your next meal or snack, think back to everything that you have already eaten during the course of your day. If you remember that you have eaten other meals or snacks that are too substantial or eaten too recently to justify taking another bite so soon, postpone eating until a later time.

While remembering what you have eaten is usually helpful, there can be a dark side to remembering what you have eaten. *The Journal of Experimental Social Psychology* has published new research that shows that people that have behaved well previously may give themselves permission to behave poorly in the future. For example, if you successfully avoid eating a brownie for breakfast, you might think, "I skipped the brownie so it's okay to have a couple of slices of pizza for lunch." In your mind, you have earned the pizzas, but you might have undermined your diet in the long run with this line of thinking.

When study participants wrote down all of the unhealthful behaviors that they had engaged in during the previous week, they failed to work as hard to meet their objectives in the following week. People that feel that they have made progress tend to feel like they have a green light to indulge themselves in unhealthful behavior.

In a second study, when people correctly dodged an unhealthful snack food, they overstated how bad the foods they avoided were in order to justify eating cookies. Thus, when people are tempted to cheat on their diets, they tend to exaggerate the "sinfulness" of the foods they did not eat in order to justify eating the bad foods that they did eat.

You may be able to counteract a tendency to justify bad behavior in three ways. First, you can view each good thing that you do as a building block towards engaging in increasingly good behavior. For example, when you turn down the brownie, use that as encouragement when you later turn down the two slices of pizza. Say to yourself, "I turned down the brownie so I clearly have the ability to turn down the pizza." Second, you can reward your own good behavior with a treat that has nothing to do with food. Perhaps there is a movie that you have been wanting to see. Now you can go out and see it in the theater as a reward for turning down that slice of cake. Third, you can reward yourself with food that you rarely get to enjoy but is health promoting. For instance, reward yourself for skipping that piece of pie by dining at your favorite swanky restaurant and ordering something good for you. The goal is to choose healthful food under all circumstances.

SECTION 4

JUST ADD YOGURT

INTRODUCTION: LEVELS OF INTENSITY

At this point, you are eating food that follows the principles of the Greek Yogurt Diet. You will want to continue to follow the Greek Yogurt Diet every step of the way in this section. We are now introducing Greek yogurt to your diet over the course of three weeks. At the same time, you will be reducing the total number of calories that you are eating. The goal is to eat as much as three cups of yogurt per day and to decrease your caloric intake enough to lose approximately 1-to-2 pounds per week.

Building on the Greek Yogurt Diet, let us explore a winning plan for incorporating yogurt as a part of your total caloric intake. We have designed a series of weeks—Week One, Week Two and Week Three—that represent increasing degrees of intensity within the Greek Yogurt Diet experience.

Think of each week as a level of intensity. Start out by following the Week One meal plan (eating yogurt throughout the day and simultaneously decreasing total calories) and then see if it places you on track to attain your health and weight loss goals. If you are moving closer to your goals, then you may simply stick with the Week One meal plan. If you are not moving closer to your weight-loss goals, then move on to the Week Two meal plan. If you are moving closer to your goals by following the meal plan of Week Two, then you may simply stick with the Week Two meal plan. If, on the other hand, you are not moving closer to your weight-loss goals, then you may move on to the Week Three meal plan.

Keep in mind that a healthy rate of weight loss is up to two pounds per week. If you find that you are losing weight much faster than two pounds per week, then go back to the meal plan of a prior week and/or increase your total daily calories so that you are losing no more than two pounds per week.

On the other hand, if you are not losing weight nearly as fast as two pounds per week, then decrease your caloric consumption or advance to the next week until you have found the level that is giving you the results that you need. We find that this first approach works best for most people.

CHAPTER 1

WEEK ONE: EAT MORE YOGURT AND REDUCE TOTAL CALORIES

Week One of the Greek Yogurt Diet involves simultaneously eating more Greek yogurt and reducing the total number of calories that you consume using portion control. Rather than eating all of your yogurt at one sitting, the idea in Week One is to eat more yogurt throughout the day. Eating yogurt as the day progresses will give you the all-day-long advantage of yogurt's ability to lower cortisol levels. You will also get all of the other benefits of Greek yogurt doled out throughout your day, rather than all at once. The goal is to eat a minimum of 2-to-4 cups of Greek yogurt per day, every day of the week. Keep in mind that the serving size of yogurt is one cup. This means that you are looking to eat 2-to-4 servings of Greek yogurt per day.

While you are eating fewer total calories, you will want to make sure that your daily caloric intake totals at least 1,600 calories if you are a woman and 1,700 calories if you are a man. Consider this a starting point. If you are not losing weight at these calorie levels, slowly reduce the amount of calories that you are consuming until you start losing weight at a healthy pace.

It has been stated by nutritionists at the Harvard School for Public Health that we should aim to eat three meals and up to two snacks per day. Distributing 1,600 or 1,700 calories evenly throughout the day helps keep your hunger at bay and your energy levels stable. Each meal should contain between 400 and 500 calories, while the snacks (up to two per day) should be around 100-to-200 calories each.

If you find that you are not losing weight at 1,600 calories a day if you are a woman or 1,700 calories a day if you are a man, then you should speak to your doctor to see if there is a medical reason why you are not losing weight. For instance, you might have a thyroid disease and, if so, you should seek out diagnosis and treatment. If there is no underlying health issue, then work with your doctor to see if you can lose weight at an even lower caloric intake in a safe and healthy way.

WEEK ONE MEAL PLAN

Day 1:

Breakfast

1 piece of fruit

1 6-ounce container of non-fat Greek yogurt (with or without fruit)

<u>Lunch</u>

1 piece grilled chicken without skin

1 serving of Fuji Apple Coleslaw with Greek Yogurt (see recipe in Section 5)

1 6-ounce container of non-fat Greek yogurt (with or without fruit)

<u>Dinner</u>

1 serving Halibut with Spicy Greek Yogurt
1 serving of side vegetables

Day 2:

<u>Breakfast</u>

2 scrambled egg whites
1 6-ounce container of non-fat Greek yogurt (with or without fruit)

<u>Lunch</u>

Beef and vegetable stew
1 6-ounce container of non-fat Greek yogurt (with or without fruit)

<u>Dinner</u>

1 serving Roast Chicken and Mango Salad with Greek Yogurt (see the recipe in Section 5)

1 serving of Pan-roasted Vegetables (see the recipe in Section 6)

Day 3:

<u>Breakfast</u>

1 apple or kiwifruit
1 6-ounce container of non-fat Greek yogurt (with or without fruit)

<u>Lunch</u>

Salad with extra virgin olive oil and vinegar dressing
1 6-ounce container of non-fat Greek yogurt (with or without fruit)

<u>Dinner</u>

1 serving Saffron Chicken Breasts with Greek Yogurt (see the recipe in Section 5)
1 serving of side vegetables

Day 4:

<u>Breakfast</u>

Pumpkin Oatmeal with Greek Yogurt (see recipe in Section 5)

<u>Lunch</u>

1 piece grilled chicken without skin
1 serving of Fuji Apple Coleslaw with Greek Yogurt (see recipe in Section 5)

<u>Dinner</u>

1 serving Creamy Curried Greek Yogurt Spinach with Tofu (see the recipe in Section 5)

1 serving of Pan-roasted Vegetables (see the recipe in Section 6)

Day 5:

Breakfast

2 scrambled egg whites
1 6-ounce container of non-fat Greek yogurt (with or without fruit)

Lunch

1 serving catfish or tilapia
1 serving of steamed vegetables
1 6-ounce container of non-fat Greek yogurt (with or without fruit)

Dinner

1 serving Curry Turkey Salad with Grapes, Cashews and Greek Yogurt (see the recipe in Section 5)
1 serving of side vegetables

Day 6:

Breakfast

1 serving Greek Yogurt Smoothie (see the recipe in Section 5)

Lunch

Beef and vegetable stew
1 6-ounce container of non-fat Greek yogurt (with or without fruit)

Dinner

1 serving Grilled Chicken in Greek Yogurt Marinade over Chopped Greek Salad (see the recipe in Section 5)

1 serving of Pan-roasted Vegetables (see the recipe in Section 6)

Day 7:

Breakfast

2 scrambled egg whites

1 6-ounce container of non-fat Greek yogurt (with or without fruit)

Lunch

1 piece grilled chicken without skin

1 serving of steamed vegetables

1 6-ounce container of non-fat Greek yogurt (with or without fruit)

Dinner

1 serving Wild Salmon atop Baby Arugula with Curried Greek Yogurt (see the recipe in Section 5)

1 serving of side vegetables

If, at the end of Week One, you are losing weight, then you may continue following the Week One meal plan. On the other hand, if you are not losing weight, then you should attempt the Week Two meal plan.

CHAPTER 2

WEEK TWO: REPLACE ONE MEAL A DAY WITH GREEK YOGURT

If you are losing up to two pounds per week by the end of Week One, you may stay at that level for as long as it proves effective. If you are not losing up to two pounds per week by the end of Week One, however, move on to Week Two. During Week Two, not only will you be eating more Greek yogurt through-out the day and, at the same time, reducing your overall caloric intake (to the same levels as you were at during Week One), you will also be replacing one meal per day with 2-to-4 cups of Greek yogurt paired with or without fruit. If you would like to pair your yogurt with fruit, we have provided a simple recipe for pairing Greek yogurt with fruit in Section 5 of this book. Alternatively, you may purchase a container that already has fruit. Depending upon how many calories you have already consumed, you will typically need to eat 2-to-4 servings of Greek yogurt in order to replace an entire meal with Greek yogurt.

Due to the fact that you will be eating so much Greek yogurt when you replace a meal with Greek yogurt, you should only be eating about 1 or 2 servings of Greek yogurt at other times over the course of your day (as opposed to the 2-to-4 cups of Greek yogurt that you were eating on a daily basis during Week 1).

I am very cautious about using meal replacements due to my experience with meal replacement shakes in the weight-loss clinic that I ran as part of my practice. I found that if meals are not satisfying, patients start to go back to their old eating habits. Based on my experience with Greek yogurt, I am confident that you will find what you are eating to be adequately substantial. This should help you to use it in place of an ordinary meal until you reach your goal. With its rich texture and feel, Greek yogurt really does give you the feeling that you have eaten a proper meal.

During Week Two, you will still be eating small amounts of Greek yogurt throughout the day, just as you were doing during Week One. Then, in addition to the Greek yogurt that you are now eating throughout the day, replace one of your meals entirely with 2-to-4 cups of Greek yogurt either with or without fruit.

One of the advantages of completely replacing a meal with yogurt is that you can maintain complete portion control for that particular meal. By eating a certain number of cups or 6-ounce containers of yogurt, for example, you will know exactly how many calories you are consuming in that meal. We typically find three, 6-ounce containers (paired with fruit) to be incredibly filling. If we find that we are still hungry, or get hungry an hour later, then we will have a fourth 6-ounce container.

You may choose which meal to replace. Generally, you will get faster results if you replace one of your larger meals with Greek yogurt rather than a smaller meal because you will be consuming fewer total calories when you take a larger meal out of the picture and replace it with Greek yogurt.

We generally recommend replacing dinner with yogurt for two reasons. First, dinner is typically one of the larger meals of the day, if not the biggest. This means that you will likely be taking in fewer total calories when you replace dinner with Greek yogurt. Second, the demands of the day are usually behind us after dinnertime. This means that we will require fewer calories from our final meal of the day, and so the fact that we have only eaten 2-to-4 cups of Greek yogurt for dinner means that the yogurt will likely give us a sufficient amount of calories to see us through until breakfast.

If hunger persists after you have replaced a meal with Greek yogurt, simply have a bit more Greek yogurt or enjoy one of the snacks suggested in Chapter 6 of Section 3 ("Snack Like a Genius"). The aim is to avoid hunger because the experience of hunger tends to lead to binge eating or giving up on the diet prematurely out of frustration.

In order to make your transition to Week Two easier, try starting out by replacing one meal a day per week, then one meal a day twice per week, etc., until you are replacing one meal a day with yogurt every single day of the week. It is okay if it takes you one or even two months to reach the point that you are able to replace one meal a day every single day of the week. The process is more like a marathon race than a sprint. The idea is to create life-long changes in our lifestyle, not to go on crash diet that will end in disappointment.

During Week Two, you may either replace the same meal each day with yogurt, such as dinner, or you may rotate the meal that you replace with Greek yogurt each day, which is typically either lunch or dinner. In the meal plan below, we rotated the meal that is replaced with yogurt, but you are free to replace the same meal each day with Greek yogurt.

WEEK TWO MEAL PLAN

Day 1:

Breakfast

2 scrambled egg whites
1 6-ounce container of non-fat Greek yogurt (with or without fruit)

Lunch

1 serving of Beef Stir-fry (see the recipe in Section 6)
1 serving of steamed vegetables

Dinner

Three 6-ounce containers of non-fat Greek yogurt (with or without fruit)

Day 2:

<u>Breakfast</u>

1 serving Spinach, Tomato and Feta Omelette (see the recipe in Section 6)

<u>Lunch</u>

1 small turkey wrap (in lettuce)
1 serving of Fuji Apple Coleslaw with Greek Yogurt (see recipe in Section 5)

<u>Dinner</u>

Three 6-ounce containers of non-fat Greek yogurt (with or without fruit)

Day 3:

<u>Breakfast</u>

2 scrambled egg whites
1 6-ounce container of non-fat Greek yogurt (with or without fruit)

<u>Lunch</u>

Three 6-ounce containers of non-fat Greek yogurt (with or without fruit)

<u>Dinner</u>

1 serving of Pan-seared Tuna with Avocado Slices and Cilantro Sauce (see the recipe in Section 6)

Day 4:

<u>Breakfast</u>

Pumpkin Oatmeal with Greek Yogurt (see recipe in Section 5)

<u>Lunch</u>

1 serving of grilled fish
1 serving of steamed vegetables

<u>Dinner</u>

Three 6-ounce containers of non-fat Greek yogurt (with or without fruit)

Day 5:

<u>Breakfast</u>

2 scrambled egg whites
1 6-ounce container of non-fat Greek yogurt (with or without fruit)

<u>Lunch</u>

1 serving of Curry Turkey Salad with Grapes, Cashews and Greek Yogurt (see the recipe in Section 5)

<u>Dinner</u>

Three 6-ounce containers of non-fat Greek yogurt (with or without fruit)

Day 6:

<u>Breakfast</u>

1 serving Greek Yogurt Smoothie (see the recipe in Section 5)

<u>Lunch</u>

Three 6-ounce containers of non-fat Greek yogurt (with or without fruit)

<u>Dinner</u>

Wild Salmon atop Baby Arugula with Curried Greek Yogurt (see the recipe in Section 5)

1 serving of Pan-roasted Vegetables (see the recipe in Section 6)

Day 7:

<u>Breakfast</u>

2 scrambled egg whites

1 6-ounce container of non-fat Greek yogurt (with or without fruit)

<u>Lunch</u>

Three 6-ounce containers of non-fat Greek yogurt (with or without fruit)

<u>Dinner</u>

1 serving of Herbed and Grass-fed Filet Mignon (see the recipe in Section 6)

1 serving of steamed vegetables

If, at the end of Week Two, you are losing weight, then you may continue following the Week Two meal plan. On the other hand, if you are not losing weight, then you should attempt the Week Three meal plan.

CHAPTER 3

WEEK THREE: MODIFIED FAST ONE DAY PER WEEK

If you are not on track to achieve your weight-loss goals during Week Two, and you have ruled out any underlying health problems, you may move on to Week Three. During Week Three, you will be eating more Greek yogurt throughout the day (at the same levels as you were eating during Week One). You will also be reducing your overall caloric intake to 1,600 calories per day if you are a woman and 1,700 calories per day if you are a man (as you did during Week One). You will now replace one meal a day every day of the week (as you did during the Week Two). Now, you will also be significantly reducing your total caloric intake once per week down to 500 calories if you are a woman and 600 calories if you are a man.

During Week Three, you will be following the meal plan of Week Two for the first six days of Week Three. Then, on the final day of Week Three, you will follow the meal plan of Week One, but you will also reduce your total caloric intake down to 500 calories if you are a woman or 600 calories if you are a man. You will not be replacing any of your meals with yogurt on the seventh day. Technically, fasting means that you are consuming nothing but water. In our plan, you will be consuming some food and so we refer to it as a modified fast.

THE FIRST SIX DAYS OF WEEK THREE

For the first six days during Week Three, you are eating as you were during Week 2. You are following the Greek Yogurt Diet and, in addition, both increasing your intake of Greek yogurt and decreasing your total caloric intake (as you did during Week 1). Also, make sure that you are replacing one meal a day with 2-to-4, 6-ounce containers of Greek yogurt paired with fruit (as you did during Week 2).

THE SEVENTH DAY OF WEEK THREE

On the seventh day of Week 3, you are following the basic Greek Yogurt Diet in terms of food choices, but the difference is that you are also reducing your total daily calories down to 500 if you are a woman and down to 600 if you are a man. You should eat a variety of foods on such "Fasting Days," and your food choices should be nutrient dense (no empty calories, please).

When you are on the Seventh Day of Week Three, you are allowed to consume your entire caloric intake (of 500 or 600 calories, depending upon your gender) in a single sitting, or by eating three small meals a day, or eating snacks over the course of your entire waking day. So far, no studies have proven that one approach to eating meals on a reduced calorie day is more helpful over another when it comes to losing weight. Breakfast might consist of an egg, one-half cup of Greek yogurt with fruit, green tea and lots of water (a minimum of eight cups per day).

For a second meal, in order to reach your daily maximum of 500 or 600 calories (depending upon your gender), you would eat some vegetables and some grilled chicken or fish. Remember to get adequate amounts of water, and as much unsweetened green tea as you like.

You may assign your Seventh Day of Week Three to a particular day, such as every Saturday or every Thursday, or you may choose your Seventh Day on the fly, completely at random. Just make sure that you never have two Fasting Days in a row.

RESEARCH ON SIGNIFICANTLY REDUCED CALORIE LEVELS

Studies have found that significantly reducing your calories can reduce insulin-like growth factor 1 (IGF-1), the hormone that has been linked to an accelerated aging process. This may mean that you will actually age at a decelerated rate due to a decrease in caloric intake.

Based on research in animal studies, it has been discovered that there are two factors that are required to make it successful. The first recommendation is that you gradually decrease your caloric intake over the course of 2.5 years. Too sharp a decrease in calories too soon may jolt your system and undermine the anti-aging benefits of fasting. A reduction in calories once per week as part of Week 3 seems like a good way to make a gradual reduction in calories. As the months progress, you may gradually reduce the calories that you consume on the fasting day, and you may eventually start to reduce your caloric intake on other days so that you are practicing a modified fast more than one day per week.

The second recommendation is that you eat foods that are nutritionally dense. By following the Greek Yogurt Diet and eating Genius Foods, you will be eating foods that will give you optimal nutrition. For more information on caloric restriction, we recommend *The 120-Year Diet* and other books by Roy L. Walford, M.D.

A significant reduction in calories also reduces blood pressure, improves lipid profiles and causes a drop in glucose levels. A drop in glucose levels can mean that you will be less likely to develop type 2 diabetes.

WEEK THREE MEAL PLAN

Day 1:

Breakfast

1 serving Spinach, Tomato and Feta Omelette (see the recipe in Section 6)

<u>Lunch</u>

1 piece grilled chicken without skin
1 serving of Fuji Apple Coleslaw with Greek Yogurt (see recipe in Section 5)

<u>Dinner</u>

Three 6-ounce containers of non-fat Greek yogurt (with or without fruit)

Day 2:

<u>Breakfast</u>

2 scrambled egg whites
1 6-ounce container of non-fat Greek yogurt (with or without fruit)

<u>Lunch</u>

1 serving of Grilled Chicken with Lemon Juice and Garlic Marinade (see the recipe in Section 6)
1 serving of steamed vegetables

<u>Dinner</u>

Three 6-ounce containers of non-fat Greek yogurt (with or without fruit)

Day 3:

<u>Breakfast</u>

2 scrambled egg whites
1 6-ounce container of non-fat Greek yogurt (with or without fruit)

<u>Lunch</u>

Three 6-ounce containers of non-fat Greek yogurt (with or without fruit)

<u>Dinner</u>

Pan-seared Tuna with Avocado Slices and Cilantro Sauce
1 serving of steamed broccoli and cauliflower

Day 4:

<u>Breakfast</u>

1 serving Greek Yogurt Smoothie (see the recipe in Section 5)

<u>Lunch</u>

1 serving of Baked Sea Bass (see the recipe in Section 6)
1 serving of Pan-roasted Vegetables (see the recipe in Section 6)

<u>Dinner</u>

Three 6-ounce containers of non-fat Greek yogurt (with or without fruit)

Day 5:

<u>Breakfast</u>

2 scrambled egg whites
1 6-ounce container of non-fat Greek yogurt (with or without fruit)

<u>Lunch</u>

Three 6-ounce containers of non-fat Greek yogurt (with or without fruit)

<u>Dinner</u>

Chili with Grass-fed Beef (see the recipe in Section 6)

1 serving of Fuji Apple Coleslaw with Greek Yogurt (see recipe in Section 5)

Day 6:

<u>Breakfast</u>

Pumpkin Oatmeal with Greek Yogurt (see recipe in Section 5)

<u>Lunch</u>

1 serving of Curry Turkey Salad with Grapes, Cashews and Greek Yogurt (see the recipe in Section 5)

<u>Dinner</u>

Three 6-ounce containers of non-fat Greek yogurt (with or without fruit)

Reduced Calorie Day 7:

<u>Breakfast</u>

2 scrambled egg whites

3-to-4 ounces of Greek yogurt

<u>A Snack</u>

One serving of any snack containing up to 100 calories (see Chapter 6 of Section 3)

<u>Dinner</u>

1 serving of grilled fish
1 serving of steamed vegetables

CHAPTER 4
ADVANCED TECHNIQUES

FINE TUNE WEEK ONE

Think of this diet as a marathon and not as a sprint. You are not trying to force yourself into a regimen that you cannot maintain and ultimately drop. The solution is to try changing things so that the Greek Yogurt Diet gives you the variety that you need. Try eating low-fat Greek yogurt instead of non-fat Greek yogurt or vice versa. Try eating regular yogurt on some days instead of Greek yogurt. Eat a Genius Food as a healthful snack when you are hungry. When you exercise, go bicycling instead of jogging or vice versa. Find what works best for you.

If you are not losing weight quickly enough during Week One, yet you do not want to move on to Week Two or Week Three, simply experiment with eating a bit more yogurt and/ or shaving a few more calories from your total caloric intake level until you find a level that starts to work for you. So, if you are a woman consuming 1,600 calories a day, try eating an extra 4 ounces of yogurt a day and dropping your total caloric intake by 50 calories down to a total of 1,550 calories a day. Wait a week or two and see if you are losing weight. If you are not losing weight at that level of reduced caloric intake, try dropping your caloric intake by another 50 calories down to 1,500 calories a day, and so forth. The key is to find the right combination of exercise, yogurt and caloric intake that works for you.

FINE TUNE WEEK TWO

You can fine tune Week Two by adjusting the meal that you replace with yogurt. If you find that you are too hungry at work after replacing your regular lunch with yogurt, try replacing dinner with Greek yogurt, instead, and go back to having your normal lunch.

Also, if you want to increase your weight loss, try replacing your largest meal of the day with yogurt. If you typically eat a huge breakfast, then replace your breakfast each day with yogurt, having smaller-sized lunches and dinners. You may also try replacing two meals a day with yogurt, although we do not recommend that you do this more than once or twice per week. Make sure that you are including some fiber in the form of fruits or vegetables when you eat Greek yogurt in place of a meal.

As you did when fine tuning Week One, try decreasing your total number of calories—50 calories at a time—until you find that you are losing at an acceptable rate (but not faster than 2 pounds per week).

FINE TUNE WEEK THREE

If you find that reducing your caloric intake one day per week is not sufficient, reduce your total caloric intake two days per week; however, you should consult with your physician to make sure that you are healthy enough before you significantly reduce your caloric intake twice per week. As we have said, make sure that your two low-calorie days are not in a row. You do not want to experience two reduced-calorie days in a row. Also, make sure that your reduction in calories is gradual.

Alternatively, if you find that reducing your caloric levels down to 500 calories if you are a woman and 600 calories if you are a man is too severe, try dropping down to only 700 calories if you are a woman and 800 calories if you are a man. The exact number of calories is up to you. Try different levels until you find the level that is right for you.

SAMPLE A VARIETY OF YOGURT PRODUCTS

Are you getting bored with your Greek yogurt selections? Try to eat as many different types and flavors of Greek yogurt available. Try popping your yogurt containers into the freezer for a little while before eating them. Try pairing your yogurt with different types of fruit. Consider eating regular, non-Greek yogurt to mix things up a bit. Try yogurt made from goat's milk.

When trying a different brand of Greek yogurt, first make sure that its product has a significant amount of whey protein.

Some manufacturers strain out the whey content in order to produce Greek yogurt. You will want to avoid such products. Unfortunately, the amount of whey protein in a given product is not printed on the label. You will need to do some research to find out how much whey protein is actually in a particular product.

FEEL FULL WITH BROTHS

Whenever we reduce the number of calories that we consume, we can miss the feeling of satiety or fullness that we used to get from our old eating habits. This feeling that we are missing out is dangerous because it can lead to binge eating or simply giving up on our new way of life.

Enter the humble broth. The volume and warmth of a broth can go a long way towards making us feel full, while it adds very few calories to our diet. You may either purchase a commercially prepared broth, or make your own following a recipe like the one found in Section 6. For health reasons, we recommend that you use as little salt as possible in your broths.

BACKING OFF

If you find a level to be too intense, give yourself permission to back off from it for a while. For instance, if you find Week Three to be too intense, stick to the meal plans for Week One or Week Two for as long as you require.

If you find that you are not losing enough weight, you can always reduce your total caloric intake while using any week's meal plan rather than moving ahead to the next week's meal plan. Simply reduce your daily caloric intake by 50 calories or 100 calories so that you will lose weight but remain at a less intense week.

Remember, also, that this process is not a sprint. It is a marathon. You want to find a pace that you can maintain for the duration of the journey. If losing two pounds per week requires too much of you, then slightly increase your caloric intake so that you are only losing one or one-and-a-half pounds per week. You have to find ways to feel comfortable with the process every step of the way because you are in it for the long haul. You will be able to enjoy the benefits of your weight loss for the rest of your life so it is okay if it takes you a little extra time to finally achieve your weight loss.

Another way to back off is to simply take a day off from yogurt from time to time, especially if eating yogurt has started to feel monotonous. You should try to substitute low-fat, high-protein foods for the yogurt that you would normally have. One of the foods that we like to eat as a replacement for yogurt on such days is sashimi (raw fish) because it is so lean yet high in protein. Having three, normal meals without any yogurt once in a while will help to cleanse your palate. Then, when you come back to yogurt the next day, it will seem slightly novel to you, helping you to stick to the Greek Yogurt Diet.

CHAPTER 5

UPON REACHING YOUR GOAL

Once you have attained your weight-loss goals, then you should make sure to do four things. First, make sure that you are getting about one hour of cardiovascular training or circuit training every single day of the week for the rest of your life, even if all you are doing is taking a brisk walk. The key is to stay active. Second, implement a meal plan similar to the one that you used in Week One, making sure that you are eating enough calories to maintain your new weight. Third, employ portion control and mindfulness while eating to make sure that you are not consuming more food than you need. Fourth, continue to consume fish oil and black tea up to 30 minutes before meals, and to drink green tea at other times throughout the day.

Be sure to send your success story to yogurtdoctor@gmail. com if you would like your personal tale to be included in a future edition of this book or if you would simply like to share it with us. We will be thrilled to hear from you and do our best to respond to each message that we receive. Also, follow @YogurtDoctor on Twitter for updates, and visit us online at www.YogurtDoctor.com.

SECTION 5

GREEK YOGURT RECIPES

BREAKFAST

GREEK YOGURT PAIRED SIMPLY WITH FRUIT

Serves 1 or 2

Ingredients

2 cups non-fat or low-fat Greek yogurt, plain

1/2 cup of fruit, whole, sliced or cubed

Sweetener, to taste (preferably honey)

Directions

1. Stir fruit into yogurt
2. Add sweetener
3. Serve in cup or bowl

GREEK YOGURT SMOOTHIE

Ingredients

1 1/2 cups frozen blueberries

3/4 cup frozen cherries

1 banana, peeled

1 cup non-fat or low-fat Greek yogurt, plain

Sweetener, to taste (preferably honey)

1/2 cup non-fat milk

1 scoop whey protein powder

5 ice cubes

Directions

1. Add all of the ingredients other than sweetener into a blender
2. Blend until smooth
3. Sweeten
4. Serve in a glass

PUMPKIN OATMEAL
WITH GREEK YOGURT

Serves 4

Ingredients

1-1/2 cups water

1/2 tsp. ground cinnamon

1 cup steel-cut oats

1/2 cup canned pumpkin puree

1 tbs. molasses

1/2 cup non-fat Greek yogurt, vanilla flavored

4 tbs. chopped walnuts, divided

Pinch of salt

Directions

1. Bring the water to a boil in a large pot; add the steel cut oats and salt; stir.
2. Reduce the heat to medium low and cook for 30 minutes; make sure you stir the oats occasionally so they do not stick to the pan
3. When the oats start to thicken, at about 30 minutes, add in the pumpkin puree and molasses
4. Stir the oats, pumpkin puree and molasses together and cook for ten more minutes
5. Spoon into 4 bowls and top each with 2 tablespoons yogurt and 1 tablespoon chopped walnuts

LUNCH & DINNER

BLACK BEAN DIP WITH GREEK YOGURT

Ingredients

1 tbs. non-fat Greek yogurt, plain

15.5-oz can black beans, drained and rinsed

2 garlic cloves, minced

2 tsp. fresh lime juice

1/4 tsp. kosher salt

Directions

1. Place beans in a medium bowl
2. Smash beans using a masher until mixture is semi-smooth
3. Stir in Greek yogurt, garlic, lime juice, and salt
4. Serve in a bowl or serving dish

CHILLED AVOCADO AND GREEK YOGURT SOUP

2 avocados, pitted and peeled

1 western yellow onion, chopped

1 cup vegetable stock

1 cup nonfat Greek yogurt

2 tbs. lemon juice

1 tsp. lemon zest

Kosher salt and freshly ground black pepper

Directions

1. In a food processor or blender, blend the avocado, onion, stock, yogurt and lemon juice, until smooth
2. Add the zest and season to taste
3. Refrigerate for one hour or until cool

CITRUS SALAD WITH GINGERED GREEK YOGURT

Ingredients

1 pink grapefruit, peeled

2 large tangerines, peeled

3 navel oranges

1/2 cup dried cranberries

2 tbs. honey

1/4 tsp ground cinnamon

16 ounces low-fat Greek yogurt, plain

2/3 cup minced crystallized ginger

1/4 cup brown sugar as a garnish

Additional dried cranberries as a garnish

Directions

To prepare fruit:

Break grapefruit and tangerines into sections; cut grapefruit sections into thirds; cut tangerine sections in half; transfer grapefruit, tangerines, and all juices to deep serving bowl; using small, sharp knife, cut all peel and white pith from oranges; slice oranges into rounds that are 1/4" thick, then cut slices into quarters; add oranges and all juices to same bowl; mix in 1/2 cup dried cranberries, honey, and cinnamon; cover and refrigerate at least 1 hour

To prepare yogurt:

Add ginger to yogurt in a bowl; whisk yogurt and ginger in a bowl until mixed

To serve:

Spoon fruit into individual bowls; spoon ginger yogurt atop fruit; sprinkle with brown sugar and dried cranberries

CREAMY CURRIED GREEK YOGURT SPINACH WITH TOFU

Serves 4

Ingredients

4 tsp. canola oil, divided

1 ounce package of firm tofu, cut into 2" cubes

3/4 tsp. of kosher salt, divided

1 western yellow onion, sliced thin in half-moons

1 red pepper, cut into 1" strips

2 cloves of garlic, finely diced

1 tsp. of fresh ginger, finely diced

1-1/2 tsp. curry powder

1/4 tsp. cumin

1 tsp. of mustard seeds

1 lb. of baby spinach

1 cup low-fat Greek yogurt, plain

Directions

1. In a medium skillet, heat 2 tsp. of oil over medium-high heat; add tofu and half of the salt; cook for 7 minutes (carefully turning every 2 minutes until lightly browned); transfer tofu to a separate plate or bowl on the side

2. Reduce heat to medium and add remaining oil to the skillet pan; add onions, garlic, red pepper, ginger and mustard seeds; cook until onion is clear (approximately 5 minutes); add spinach a handful at a time and cook until it wilts

3. In a small bowl, mix together yogurt, curry, cumin and remaining salt; heat yogurt by adding some of the spinach mixture until it is warm throughout; add yogurt to skillet; then add tofu; reduce heat to low and stir carefully for 2 minutes

CURRIED GREEK YOGURT

Ingredients

2/3 tsp. large shallot, finely diced

2/3 tsp. cider vinegar

2/3 tsp. kosher salt

1/3 tsp. curry powder

1 pinch cayenne

1 pinch sugar

2/3 cup low-fat Greek yogurt, plain

Directions

1. Place yogurt in a small bowl
2. Combine shallot, vinegar, salt, curry, cayenne, sugar and yogurt

CURRY TURKEY SALAD WITH GRAPES, CASHEWS AND GREEK YOGURT

Serves 4

2 tbs. reduced-fat sour cream

2 tbs. low-fat Greek yogurt, plain

1 tbs. fresh lime juice

1 tbs. honey

1 tsp. curry powder

1/4 tsp. salt

1/4 tsp. freshly ground black pepper

2 cups skinless, free-range turkey, cooked and chopped

1 cup seedless red grapes, halved

1/2 cup diced celery

1/4 cup chopped western yellow onion

2 tbs. cashew pieces

1 head butter lettuce (or, boston bibb) or iceberg lettuce

Directions

1. Combine sour cream, yogurt, lime juice, honey, curry powder, salt and pepper in a large bowl

2. Add turkey, grapes, celery, onion, and cashews; stir gently to combine

3. Serve on plates in lettuce wraps

DILL DIP WITH GREEK YOGURT

Ingredients

2 cups nonfat Greek yogurt

3 tbs. fresh chopped dill

1 tsp. minced fresh garlic

Kosher salt and pepper

Vegetables for dipping

Direction

1. Place yogurt, dill and garlic into a food processor or blender
2. Blend for 60 seconds
3. Season with salt and pepper to taste
4. Blend until smooth
5. Refrigerate before serving

FUJI APPLE COLESLAW
WITH GREEK YOGURT

Serves 8

Ingredients
8 cups mixed red and green cabbage, shredded
1 12-ounce bag broccoli slaw mix
1/2 cup shredded carrots
1/2 cup thinly sliced scallions
1-1/2 cups Greek Yogurt "Mayonnaise" (see recipe in this
section)
2 tbs. distilled white vinegar
1 tbs. fresh lemon juice
1 tsp. grated garlic
Kosher salt, to taste
Freshly ground pepper, to taste
1 fuji apple, cored (Granny Smith apple, optionally)

Directions
To make slaw:
Combine red and green cabbages, broccoli slaw, carrots, and
scallions in a large bowl; mix thoroughly

To make dressing:
Whisk Greek Yogurt "Mayonnaise," vinegar, lemon juice, and
garlic in a medium bowl until smooth; season with salt and
pepper; keep dressing separate until serving

To prepare apple and then combine slaw and dressing:
Immediately before serving, cut core from apple and cut
apple into matchstick-size sticks; add apple to slaw mixture
and toss to evenly incorporate; add dressing and toss to coat
the slaw evenly

GODDESS DIP OR DRESSING
WITH GREEK YOGURT

Ingredients

1 chopped avocado

2 garlic cloves, minced

2 scallions, chopped

1/4 cup fresh basil, chopped

1 tbs. minced fresh tarragon leaves

1/4 cup low-fat Greek yogurt, plain

1/4 cup white wine vinegar

1-1/2 tbs. lemon juice

Extra virgin olive oil (enough to turn dip into dressing with desired amount)

Salt, to taste

Directions

1. Combine the avocado, garlic, scallions, basil, parsley and tarragon and then blend in a food processor

2. Add the Greek yogurt, white wine vinegar and lemon juice in the processor

3. Process until smooth

4. Serve with vegetables that have a low glycemic index (such as broccoli, carrots and cauliflower) as a dip or drizzle over steamed vegetables

5. To turn this dip into a dressing, add olive oil 1/4 cup at a time, processing constantly until you have reached the desired amount of consistency; toss with salad greens

GREEK YOGURT "MAYONNAISE"

Ingredients

4 large garlic cloves

1 tsp. extra virgin olive oil

3/4 cup Greek yogurt, plain

2 tbs. mayonnaise

1 tbs. Dijon mustard

1 tbs. lemon juice

Salt and pepper, to taste

Directions

1. Place garlic unpeeled in a dish with olive oil, microwave on high for 1 to 1-1/2 minutes until very soft
2. Squeeze garlic from skin into a bowl; mash with a fork until smooth
3. Add Greek yogurt, mayonnaise, Dijon mustard, lemon juice, salt and pepper to taste
4. Stir well until fully blended
5. Will keep in a refrigerator for up to three days

GRILLED CHICKEN IN GREEK YOGURT MARINADE OVER CHOPPED GREEK SALAD

Serves 2

Ingredients
2 large chicken breasts
Wooden skewers soaked in water for one hour
1 cup low-fat, Greek yogurt, plain
Four cloves garlic
Juice of 1 lemon
6 roma (or, plum) tomatoes, diced
1 small cucumber: peeled, quartered lengthwise, and chopped
3 western yellow onions, chopped
1/4 cup fresh basil leaves, cut into thin strips
3 tablespoons extra virgin olive oil
2 tablespoons balsamic vinegar
3 tablespoons crumbled feta cheese
Kosher salt and freshly ground black pepper, to taste

Directions
To prepare marinated chicken and marinade reserve:
1. Mix together yogurt, garlic and lemon juice to make marinade
2. Reserve 2 oz. of mixture in a separate bowl
3. Cut up chicken into one-inch chunks

224

4. Toss chicken with marinade
5. Cover and store marinade in refrigerator for at least 2 hours

To prepare salad:
1. In a large bowl, toss together the tomatoes, cucumber, onions, basil, olive oil, balsamic vinegar, and feta cheese
2. Season with salt and pepper to taste

To grill chicken:
1. Skewer chicken
2. Grill chicken 2-1/2 minutes on each side

To serve:
1. Spread reserve marinade over cooked chicken
2. Place chicken skewers over salad

GRILLED EGGPLANT WITH GREEK YOGURT DRESSING

Ingredients

1 pound small eggplants

1 medium minced, fresh western yellow onion, divided

3 minced garlic cloves, divided

1-1/2 cups low-fat Greek yogurt, plain

1/4 tsp. salt

1/4 tsp. freshly ground black pepper

1/8 tsp. cayenne pepper

Directions

1. Cut the eggplants in half (lengthwise) up to the stem; do not cut through

2. Spread about 2/3 of the onion and garlic between the eggplant halves, and press the two sides back together

3. Grill the eggplants, turning once or twice, until they are blackened and collapsed, 10-15 minutes; a little burning is acceptable

4. Meanwhile, mix the remaining onion and garlic with the yogurt; then season with salt, black pepper, and cayenne

5. When cooked, let the eggplants cool a bit, then peel off the skins and let cool further; roughly chop the eggplants, reserving any juices, then mix with the yogurt dressing; serve at room temperature

MASHED CAULIFLOWER
WITH GREEK YOGURT

Ingredients

1 head of cauliflower (florets but no stems)

1 6-ounce container of Greek yogurt, plain

2 tbs. canola butter (see the recipe in Section 6)

3 tbs. grated parmigiano

2 cloves of garlic, chopped

1/2 small shallot, chopped

1 chopped scallion, for garnish

Salt, pepper and seasonings, to taste

Directions

1. In a medium pot, bring water to boil
2. Add cauliflower florets to the boiling water and let cook for 8 minutes or until soft
3. Remove and drain
4. In a food processor, combine the cauliflower with the Greek yogurt, canola butter, garlic and shallots and then blend until you achieve a creamy consistency
5. Add salt, pepper and other seasoning, to taste, and blend until mixed in
6. Transfer to a bowl and, while hot, mix in the parmigiano
7. Top with scallions for garnish

MEXICALI AVOCADO DIP
WITH GREEK YOGURT

Ingredients

1 cup non-fat Greek yogurt, plain

1 tsp. fresh lime juice

2 ripe avocados, halved, pitted, peeled, and chopped

½ jalapeño, halved, seeded, and finely chopped

½ tsp. ground cumin

Kosher salt, to taste

Directions

1. In a medium bowl, mash avocados
2. Add Greek yogurt, jalapeño, cumin, kosher salt (to taste) and lime juice to avocados
3. Mash all ingredients together
4. Serve as part of a Mexican dish in place of guacamole or as a dip

MINT RAITA

Ingredients

1 cup low-fat Greek yogurt, plain

3 tbs. fresh mint, chopped

2 tbs. fresh cilantro, chopped

1-1/4 tsp. freshly grated lime zest

Kosher salt, to taste

Freshly ground pepper, to taste

Directions

1. Mix yogurt, mint, cilantro, and lime peel in small bowl
2. Season with salt and pepper
3. Cover; then chill until cold
4. Serve as a sauce or dip with meat and/or vegetable dishes

HALIBUT WITH SPICY
GREEK YOGURT

Ingredients

24 ounces skinless halibut fillet 1 1/4" thick, cut
into 4 portions

3/4 tsp. salt

1/4 tsp. black pepper

1/4 cup extra virgin olive oil

Spicy Greek Yogurt (see the recipe in this Section)

Directions

1. Put fish in a plate and sprinkle salt and pepper
   all over fish

2. Heat oil in a 12-inch heavy skillet over
   moderately high heat until hot but not
   smoking

3. Sauté fish, turning over once, until golden and
   just cooked through, 5-to-7 minutes total

4. Serve fish with each piece going onto an
   individual plate with spicy yogurt on the side

PENNE WITH WILD MUSHROOMS AND GREEK YOGURT

Serves 2

Ingredients

2 tbs. extra virgin olive oil

3 shallots, peeled and finely chopped

2 cloves garlic, peeled and crushed

2/3 lbs. wild mushrooms, fresh, wiped and sliced

1 tbs. balsamic vinegar

1 box Barilla PLUS® penne

¼ tsp. freshly grated nutmeg

Kosher salt and freshly ground black pepper, to taste

2 6 oz. containers of nonfat Greek yogurt

2 tbs. freshly chopped basil and parsley

Directions

1. Heat olive oil in a large saucepan; sauté the chopped shallots and crushed garlic for 2-3 minutes; stir in the mushrooms, add vinegar and cook for another 4 minutes

2. Cook the penne according to the pack instructions

3. Stir the pasta into the mushrooms and reheat; season with salt and pepper; add the Greek yogurt and stir well; garnish with fresh herbs

POTATO SKINS TOPPED WITH GREEK YOGURT AND CHIVES

Serves 8

Ingredients

8 (3-inch-long) russet potatoes (about 2 1/4 pounds), scrubbed and thoroughly dried

2 tablespoons canola butter (see the recipe in Section 6), melted

Kosher salt

Freshly ground black pepper

2 cups shredded sharp, light (reduced fat) cheddar cheese (about 4 ounces)

1/3 cup low-fat Greek yogurt, plain

2 tbs. finely chopped fresh chives

Directions

1. Heat the oven to 400 °F and arrange a rack in the middle
2. Pierce each potato several times with a fork or sharp knife
3. Place the potatoes directly on the oven rack and bake until the skins are crisp and a knife easily pierces the potatoes (about 45-to-50 minutes)
4. Transfer to a wire rack until cool enough to handle, about 10 minutes
5. Set the oven to broil.
6. Slice each potato in half lengthwise to produce 16 potato skins

7. Using a spoon, scoop out the flesh, leaving about 1/4 inch intact
8. Brush the insides of the potatoes with the butter and season with salt and pepper
9. Flip the potatoes over, brush the skin sides with the butter, and season with salt and pepper
10. Evenly space the potato halves skin-side up on a baking sheet and broil until the butter foams and the skins start to crisp, about 2 to 3 minutes (make sure they do not burn)
11. Flip the potato halves over and broil until the top edges just start to brown, about 2 to 3 minutes more
12. Fill each skin with cheese
13. Place in the broiler and broil until the cheese is melted and bubbling, about 4 to 5 minutes
14. Remove from the broiler and top each with 1 teaspoon of the sour cream and a sprinkling of the chives

RANCH DRESSING WITH GREEK YOGURT

Ingredients

1 cup Greek yogurt, plain

1 envelope ranch dressing mix

¼ cup milk

Directions

1. Combine yogurt and mix
2. Whisk in milk until thoroughly combined
3. Pour into a jar or plastic bottle and refrigerate for 4 hours
4. May be stored in refrigerator

ROAST CHICKEN AND MANGO SALAD WITH GREEK YOGURT

Ingredients

3 tbs. extra virgin olive oil

2 tbs. purchased mango chutney, large pieces finely chopped

1 tbs. fresh lemon juice

1 tbs. curry powder

Kosher salt, to taste

Freshly ground pepper, to taste

1-1/2 tsp. water

5-ounce package arugula

3-1/2-pound free-range, roast chicken, boned, meat coarsely shredded into bite-size pieces

1 large mango, peeled, pitted, sliced or 2 large peaches, halved, pitted, sliced

1 cup non-fat Greek yogurt, plain

Directions

1. Whisk first 4 ingredients and 1-1/2 teaspoons water in small bowl and blend into dressing
2. Add more water by teaspoonfuls if dressing is too thick
3. Season dressing to taste with salt and pepper
4. Place arugula in large bowl
5. Add half of dressing and toss to coat
6. Divide arugula among plates
7. Mingle cooked chicken together with mango over each serving
8. Drizzle with remaining dressing
9. Top each serving with dollop of yogurt

SAFFRON CHICKEN BREASTS WITH GREEK YOGURT

Serves 4

Ingredients

1-1/2 cups low-fat Greek yogurt, plain

1 pinch saffron threads, crushed

1 garlic clove, minced

4 (6-ounce) skinless, boneless free-range chicken breast halves

Kosher salt, to taste

Freshly ground pepper, to taste

Directions

1. Preheat broiler
2. Combine yogurt, approximately 1/2 tsp. salt, approximately 1/8 tsp. pepper, a pinch of saffron, and garlic in a large bowl
3. Add chicken, tossing to coat
4. Let stand at room temperature for 15 minutes
5. Place chicken on a broiler pan coated with canola oil cooking spray
6. Broil for 10 minutes per side, or until the chicken is cooked through and the surface is browned

SAVORY CHOPPED SALAD WITH GREEK YOGURT

Serves 4

Ingredients

8 ounces low-fat Greek yogurt, plain

1 medium cucumber, peeled and chopped

2 tbs. chopped red onion

1/2 tsp. kosher salt

1/2 tsp. freshly ground black pepper

8 halves oil-packed dried tomatoes, finely chopped

Directions

Combine ingredients in a bowl and mix well by stirring

SPICY GREEK YOGURT

Ingredients

1 cup low-fat, Greek yogurt, plain

1/2 cucumber, peeled, seeded, and finely diced

2 tbs. chopped fresh dill

1 tbs. finely chopped onion

1 tbs. fresh lemon juice

2 tsp. dried maras pepper

1/2 tsp. kosher salt

Directions

1. Place the yogurt in a large mixing bowl

2. Mix in all of the other ingredients until blended

STUFFED MUSHROOMS WITH GREEK YOGURT

Ingredients

20 medium mushrooms

1/2 cup low-fat Greek yogurt, plain

1/4 cup western yellow onion, chopped

2 cloves garlic, chopped

1 tbs. extra virgin olive oil

1 tbs. balsamic vinegar

1/2 tsp. teriyaki sauce

2 cups fresh baby spinach, chopped

Kosher salt and pepper, to taste

Directions

1. Wash the mushrooms and carefully remove the stems keeping the heads intact
2. Finely chop the stems
3. Pour the oil into a small skillet or saucepan and heat until warm
4. Add the onions, garlic and vinegar; cook for 1 to 2 minutes
5. Add the chopped mushroom stems and teriyaki sauce and cook, stirring occasionally, for 3 to 5 minutes, until the mushrooms soften
6. Add the spinach and cook, continuing to stir, until the leaves are wilted and the liquid in the pan is absorbed
7. Remove from the heat; let cool for a few minutes, then stir in the yogurt

8. Season with salt and pepper to taste

9. Preheat the oven to 350 °F.

10. Stuff the spinach filling into the mushroom caps

11. Place the mushrooms in a baking pan and bake for 20 minutes, until tender

12. Remove from the oven and let sit for a few minutes for the filling to set before serving

TOASTED QUINOA WITH GREEK YOGURT

Ingredients

1/2 tbs. of raw black or red quinoa

5 raw pistachios, shelled, raw, unsalted and roughly chopped

5 raw almonds, unsalted and roughly chopped

1/2 cup of Greek yogurt

2 medjool dates, pitted and chopped

1/2 tsp. of fresh lemon zest

Kosher salt, to taste

Extra virgin olive oil

Directions

1. Add the quinoa to a dry skillet over medium heat; toast the quinoa, stirring occasionally, until it begins to pop; once it starts popping, transfer it to a small bowl and set aside

2. Add the chopped nuts to the same skillet and carefully toast, stirring occasionally, until they begin to let off an aroma; watch closely so as not to burn the nuts; when toasted, transfer the nuts to a small bowl

3. Scoop the yogurt into the center of a plate. Sprinkle with nuts, quinoa, dates, and a pinch of salt. Toss on some lemon zest, and give the dish a light drizzle of olive oil

TOMATO SOUP WITH GREEK YOGURT

Serves 6

Ingredients

1/2 cup Greek yogurt, plain

1 tbs. extra virgin olive oil

1/2 cup western yellow onion, chopped

2 cloves garlic, minced

3 15-oz. cans diced tomatoes

15 oz. Vegetable Broth (use recipe in Section 6 or commercially prepared broth)

1 tsp. sugar

1/4 cup chopped fresh basil

Dash of crushed red pepper flakes

Kosher salt and freshly ground black pepper, to taste

Directions

1. In a large pot, heat the olive oil over medium heat; add the onion and garlic and cook until tender, about 5 minutes; stir in the bay leaves; add the tomatoes and vegetable broth; stir in sugar and fresh basil; season with red pepper flakes, salt, and pepper, to taste; simmer for 15 minutes.

2. Blend the soup in a standing blender and return to the pot; stir in the Greek yogurt until well combined.

WALDORF SALAD WITH GREEK YOGURT "MAYONNAISE"

Serves 4

Ingredients

2/3 cup Greek yogurt "mayonnaise" (see the recipe in this Section)

2 tsp. lemon juice

1/4 tsp. kosher salt

3 cups cooked, free-range chicken breast, chopped

1 medium red apple, diced

1 cup red or green grapes, halved

1 cup sliced celery

1/2 cup walnuts, chopped and divided (may be toasted)

Directions

1. Whisk "mayonnaise," lemon juice and salt in a large bowl
2. Add chicken, apple, grapes, celery and 1/4 cup walnuts
3. Stir to coat well
4. Top with the remaining 1/4 cup walnuts

WILD SALMON ATOP BABY ARUGULA WITH CURRIED GREEK YOGURT

Serves 2

Ingredients

2 center-cut filets of wild salmon (6 oz. each) (Atlantic salmon, optionally)

1-1/2 tbs. fresh lemon juice

1-1/2 tbs. extra virgin olive oil

Kosher salt, to taste

Freshly ground black pepper, to taste

Curried Greek Yogurt (see the recipe in this Section)

For salad:

3 cups baby arugula leaves

2/3 cup grape or cherry tomatoes, halved

1/4 cup thinly slivered red onion

Kosher salt, to taste

Freshly ground black pepper, to taste

1 tbs. extra virgin olive oil

1 tbs. red-wine vinegar

Directions

1. Place the salmon fillets in a shallow bowl; toss well with lemon juice, olive oil, salt and pepper; let rest for 15 minutes

2. Cook the salmon, skin-side down, in a nonstick skillet over medium-high heat for 2-to-3 minutes, shaking the pan and carefully lifting the salmon with a spatula to

loosen it from the pan; reduce the heat to medium. Cover the pan and cook until the salmon is cooked through, 3-to-4 minutes more; the skin should be crisp and the flesh medium rare

3. Meanwhile, combine the arugula, tomatoes and onion in a bowl; just before serving, season with salt and pepper and drizzle with oil and vinegar; toss well

4. Place salmon over arugula and top with Curried Greek Yogurt (see the recipe in this Section)

DESSERT

GREEK YOGURT "ICE POPS"

Ingredients

1 cup of ripe berries (single type of berry or combination)

1 cup of non-fat Greek yogurt, plain

Fresh mint, to taste

Lemons, to taste

Sugar, to taste

Directions

1. Fill food processor or blender with ripe berries and yogurt
2. Blend until smooth
3. Add mint, lemons and sugar as you blend until you obtain desired sweetness and taste
4. Pour mixture into a clean, ice-cube tray
5. Place in freezer
6. Poke toothpicks into center of each cube as mixture freezes

GRILLED FRUIT WITH HONEYED GREEK YOGURT SAUCE

Ingredients

Wooden skewers soaked in water for one hour

8 firm yet ripe plums, each cut into 8 wedges

4 firm yet ripe peeled peaches, each cut into 8 wedges

Honeyed Greek Yogurt Sauce (see the recipe in this Section)

Directions

1. Prepare grill for cooking
2. Pierce 4 pieces of fruit with each skewer
3. When fire is medium-hot, grill fruit in batches on lightly oiled grill rack, turning once, until browned and slightly softened, 2.5 minutes each side
4. Serve fruit on skewers with Honeyed Greek Yogurt Sauce on the side

HOMEMADE FROZEN GREEK YOGURT

Ingredients

1/4 cup water

2/3 cup sugar

2 egg whites, room temperature

3-1/2 cups nonfat Greek yogurt, cold

2 tsp. vanilla extract

1. In a small saucepan, combine water and sugar; bring to a boil over medium-high heat; when sugar comes to a full boil, continue to boil for 1.5 minutes

2. While the sugar boils, beat egg whites to soft peaks in a large, clean bowl; when the sugar is ready, continue beating the eggs at a low speed and very slowly stream in the hot sugar; when all the sugar has been incorporated, turn up mixer to high and beat until meringue is glossy and has cooled down to almost room temperature

3. Fold cold yogurt and vanilla into the meringue

4. Freeze yogurt mixture in ice cream maker

HONEYED GREEK
YOGURT SAUCE

12 oz (1-1/2 cups) non-fat Greek yogurt, plain

3 tbs. honey

2 tbs. fresh lime juice

3 tbs. finely chopped fresh mint

Directions

1. Place yogurt in a small bowl
2. Stir together yogurt, honey, lime juice, and mint in a small bowl
3. Chill until ready to serve

SECTION 6

MORE RECIPES

BREAKFAST

SPINACH, TOMATO AND FETA OMELETTE

Serves 1-2

Ingredients

8 egg whites

1 cup baby spinach, chopped

1/4 tsp. dried oregano

Salt, to taste

1 roma (plum) tomato, sliced

2 tbs. feta cheese, crumbled

1/4 western yellow onion, thinly sliced

Directions

1. Pour egg whites into a medium bowl with spinach, oregano and salt

2. Beat until well blended

3. Lightly coat a 9-inch, nonstick skillet with cooking spray

4. Heat over medium heat

5. Pour egg whites, spinach, oregano and salt into skillet

6. Cook until bottom is lightly browned and firm, about 5-6 minutes

7. With a spatula, flip the omelet to the other side and cook 3 minutes more

8. Transfer omelet to a platter

9. Sprinkle tomatoes, onions and cheese on one half and fold over other half to cover

LUNCH & DINNER

BABA GANOUSH

Ingredients

1 large eggplant (about 450 grams)

1 glove garlic, pressed

1/4 tsp. kosher salt, plus extra

1/4 cup parsley, finely chopped, plus extra for garnish

2 tbs. tahini (or, sesame paste), including oil

2 tbs. lemon juice

Directions

1. Preheat oven to 450 °F.
2. Prick eggplant with a fork and place on a cookie sheet lined with foil
3. Bake the eggplant until it is soft inside, about 20 to 30 minutes; let the eggplant cool
4. Cut the eggplant in half lengthwise
5. Drain off the liquid and scoop the pulp into a food processor fitted with the blade attachment
6. Add the rest of the ingredients and process to a paste consistency
7. Season with more salt, to taste
8. Garnish with extra parsley
9. Serve as a dip with fresh vegetables

BAKED SEA BASS

Serves 4

Ingredients

2 lbs. sea bass, cleaned and scaled, cut into 4 portions

6 garlic cloves, crushed

2 tbs. extra virgin olive oil

2 tbs. fresh parsley leaves

4 tsp. fresh coarse ground black pepper

2 tsp. kosher salt

4 lemon wedges

Directions

1. Preheat oven to 450 °F
2. In a cup, mix garlic, oil, salt and pepper
3. Place fish in shallow, glass bakeware
4. Carefully brush all sides of fish with oil mix
5. Bake fish, uncovered, for 15 minutes
6. Sprinkle with parsley
7. Continue to bake for 5 more minutes
8. Drizzle remaining pan juices over fish and garnish with lemon wedges

BAKED TOMATOES

Serves 2

Ingredients

2 small tomatoes, cut into 1/2-inch-thick slices

Extra virgin olive oil

2 tbs. western yellow onions, chopped

1 tsp. garlic, minced

1/4 tsp. sugar

Kosher salt, to taste

Freshly ground pepper, to taste

1 tbs. freshly grated Romano cheese

1 tbs. fresh basil, shredded

1 tsp. fresh oregano, chopped

Directions

1. Preheat oven to 350 °F
2. Arrange tomato slices in an 11" x 7" inch baking dish coated with olive oil
3. Sprinkle tomato slices with green onions, garlic, sugar, salt and pepper
4. Bake for 10 minutes
5. Remove from oven
6. Top tomato slices with a sprinkle of cheese, basil, and oregano
7. Serve warm

BEEF STIR-FRY

Serves 4

Ingredients

1 pound grass-fed, top sirloin or chuck steaks (about 1/2 inch thick), trimmed

1 large garlic clove, minced

3 tbs. canola oil

2 medium bell peppers, one red, one green, sliced into 1/4-inch strips

1/2 western yellow onion, thinly sliced lengthwise (root to top)

1 dozen cherry tomatoes, cut in half

2 tbs. chopped cilantro (or, coriander)

1 tbs. teriyaki sauce

2 tsp. sesame oil

Kosher salt and freshly ground black pepper, to taste

Directions

1. Season the steaks with salt and pepper and rub minced garlic over one side; place the steaks between two sheets of plastic wrap; with a meat pounder, pound the steaks to a 1/4 inch thickness; let the steaks sit for 10 minutes to absorb the flavor of the garlic; then cut them across the grain in 1/2-inch wide strips

2. Heat 2 tbs. of oil in a large skillet on high heat; add the sliced onions and bell peppers, cook, stirring, until just

barely tender, about 1-2 minutes; remove the vegetables
from the pan to a bowl and keep warm

3. Heat an additional tbs. of oil in the skillet on high heat,
    until the oil is shimmering, but not smoking; add the
    strips of beef let the beef brown initially, without stirring,
    but as soon as it is brown on one side, then stir; cook
    for no more than 1-1/2 minutes; add the peppers and
    onions, tomatoes, cilantro, soy sauce and 2 tsp. canola oil
    and cook for a half minute longer, stirring; remove from
    heat

4. Add salt and pepper to taste

CANOLA BUTTER

Ingredients

1 stick butter

1/2 cup canola oil

Directions

1. Bring oil and butter sticks to room temperate
2. In a blender, combine ingredients and blend until smooth and creamy
3. Use a spatula around the top edge in the blender while the mixture is blending to thoroughly combine the oil and butter
4. Pour mixture into bowl with lid
5. Refrigerate several hours
6. Use in place of butter

CHICKEN CACCIATORE

Serves 4

Ingredients

2 tsp. extra virgin olive oil

4 boneless, skinless free-range chicken-breast halves

kosher salt, to taste

freshly ground black pepper, to taste

1 small yellow or green bell pepper, cut into thin strips

2 cups sliced crimini mushrooms

1/2 cup dry red wine

1-1/2 cups tomato-and-basil pasta sauce, homemade or store-bought

2 tbs. chopped fresh parsley

Directions

1. Heat oil in large nonstick skillet over medium-high heat; add chicken
2. Sprinkle approximately 1/2 tsp. salt and pepper over chicken; cook 4 minutes per side
3. Transfer chicken to a plate; set aside
4. Combine bell pepper and mushrooms in skillet over medium heat. Sprinkle approximately 1/4 tsp. salt
5. Cook 4 minutes, stirring occasionally
6. Add wine; cook 2 minutes
7. Stir in sauce; heat through
8. Return chicken to skillet; reduce heat and simmer, turning once, 4 minutes or until cooked through
9. Plate chicken cacciatore
10. Place parsley atop each plate

CHILI WITH GRASS-FED BEEF

Ingredients

2 pounds lean, grass-fed beef, ground

1 (46 fluid ounce) can tomato juice

1 (29 ounce) can tomato sauce

1 (15 ounce) can kidney beans, drained and rinsed

1 (15 ounce) can pinto beans, drained and rinsed

1 1/2 cups chopped onion

1/4 cup chopped green bell pepper

1/8 tsp. ground cayenne pepper

1/2 tsp. sugar

1/2 tsp. dried oregano

1/2 tsp. ground black pepper

1 tsp. kosher salt

1-1/2 tsp. ground cumin

1/4 cup chili powder

Ingredients

1. Place ground beef in a large, deep skillet
2. Cook over medium-high heat until evenly brown; drain and crumble
3. In a large pot over high heat combine the ground beef, tomato juice, tomato sauce, kidney beans, pinto beans, onions, bell pepper, cayenne pepper, sugar, oregano, ground black pepper, salt, cumin and chili powder
4. Bring to a boil, then reduce heat to low
5. Simmer for 1-1/2 hours

(If using a slow cooker, set on low, add ingredients, and cook for 8 to 10 hours.)

CURRIED WILD SALMON

Serves 6

Ingredients

1/3 cup soy sauce

1/2 cup canola oil

1 tsp. garlic powder

1 tsp. curry powder

1 tsp. lemon-pepper seasoning

1 tsp. Worcestershire sauce

6 wild salmon (Atlantic salmon, optionally) fillets
(8 ounces each)

Directions

1. In a large, resealable plastic bag, combine 1/3 cup of canola oil, the soy sauce, garlic powder, curry powder, lemon-pepper, Worcestershire sauce
2. Add the salmon
3. Seal bag and turn to coat; refrigerate for 1 hour
4. Drain and discard marinade
5. Using long-handled tongs, moisten a paper towel with the remainder of the canola oil and lightly coat the grill rack
6. Place salmon skin side down on rack
7. Grill, covered, over medium heat or broil 4 in. from the heat for 10-12 minutes or until fish flakes easily with a fork

EDAMAME, BLACK BEANS AND BLACK-EYED PEAS SALAD

Serves 6

Ingredients

1-1/2 cups frozen shelled edamame (8 ounces)

1/4 cup extra virgin olive oil

1 teaspoon ground cumin

1 (15-ounce) can black beans, drained and rinsed

1 (15-ounce) can black-eyed peas, drained and rinsed

1/2 cup chopped red onion

2 cups thinly sliced celery

2 tbs. fresh lime juice

1/2 cup chopped fresh cilantro (or, coriander)

1 tsp. finely chopped garlic

1-1/2 tsp. salt

1/4 tsp. black pepper

Directions

1. Cook edamame in a 1-1/2 to 2 quart saucepan of boiling salted water, uncovered, 4 minutes

2. Drain in a colander; then rinse under cold water to stop cooking

3. Heat oil in a small heavy skillet over moderately low heat until hot but not smoking

4. Cook cumin by dropping cumin into oil, stirring, until fragrant and a shade darker, about 30 seconds, producing cumin oil

5. Pour cumin oil into a large bowl that will not be damaged by the heat of the cumin oil

6. Add edamame and remaining ingredients to cumin oil and toss to coat

7. Let stand 10 minutes for flavors to blend

GREEN BEAN, WATERCRESS AND WALNUT SALAD

Serves 10

Ingredients

12 ounces green beans, trimmed, halved diagonally (about 3 cups)

1/4 cup red wine vinegar

1-1/2 tbs. Dijon mustard

1/2 cup extra virgin olive oil

4 bunches watercress, trimmed

1-1/2 cups walnuts, toasted, coarsely chopped (about 6 ounces)

1-1/2 cups cherry tomatoes, halved

Salt and freshly ground pepper, to taste

Directions

1. Cook beans in large pot of boiling salted water until crisp-tender, about 4 minutes
2. Drain the beans
3. Transfer beans to large bowl of ice water to cool
4. Drain the beans; pat dry
5. Whisk vinegar and mustard in a small bowl to blend
6. Gradually whisk in olive oil
7. Season with salt and pepper
8. Combine beans, watercress, walnuts and tomatoes in large bowl
9. Toss with enough vinaigrette to coat
10. Season to taste with salt and pepper

GRILLED CHICKEN MARINATED IN LEMON JUICE AND GARLIC

Serves 6

Ingredients

2 tbs. extra virgin olive oil

3 tbs. fresh lemon juice

2 garlic cloves, minced

6 (6-ounce) skinless, boneless chicken breast halves

1/2 tsp. kosher salt

1/2 tsp. freshly ground black pepper

Cooking spray

Directions

1. Combine first 4 ingredients in a large zip-top plastic bag; seal
2. Marinate in refrigerator 45 minutes, turning occasionally
3. Take chicken out of bag; discard marinade
4. Sprinkle chicken evenly with salt and pepper
5. Prepare grill to medium-high heat
6. Place chicken on grill rack coated with cooking spray
7. Grill 6 minutes on each side or until done.

GRILLED VEGETABLES MARINATED IN HONEYED BALSAMIC VINAIGRETTE

Serves 2-to-4

Ingredients

Wooden skewers soaked in water for one hour

1 portabello mushroom

1 red pepper

10 stalks of asparagus

1 squash

1 zucchini

1 western yellow onion

1/4 cup extra virgin olive oil

2 tbs. honey

1 tbs. dark balsamic vinegar

1 clove garlic, minced

1 tbs. fresh thyme

Parmigiano, shaved

Directions

1. Cut tofu and veggies into 1 1/2 inch chunks
2. Pour veggies into large, re-sealable plastic bag
3. Add marinade and toss to mix
4. Seal bag and turn to coat; refrigerate for 1 hour
5. Marinate for at least two hours or overnight
6. Drain and discard marinade
7. Thread veggies onto skewers
8. Grill veggies
9. Put veggies on serving tray or plates
10. Immediately top with parmigiano

HALIBUT WITH HERBS AND CAPERS

Serves 4

1/4 cup western yellow onion, chopped

1/4 cup fresh parsley leaves

1 tbs. fresh cilantro (or, coriander) leaves

2 tsp. lemon zest, freshly grated

1 tbs. lemon juice, juiced

1 tbs. green olives, chopped and pitted

2 tsp. drained capers, rinsed

1 clove garlic, minced

1/8 tsp. freshly ground pepper

Kosher salt, to taste

2 tbs. extra virgin olive oil

1 1-pound halibut fillet, cut into 4 portions

Directions

1. Place onion, parsley, cilantro, lemon zest, lemon juice, olives, capers, garlic, and pepper in a food processor; pulse several times to chop

2. Add oil and process, scraping down the sides several times, until a pesto-like paste forms

3. Rub halibut with salt, to taste

4. Top halibut with the herb paste

5. Cover and refrigerate for 30 minutes

6. Preheat oven to 450 °F

7. Coat a 7-by-11-inch baking dish with canola cooking spray

8. Arrange the halibut in the dish and spoon any extra herb mixture on top

9. Bake, uncovered, until the fish is opaque in the center, 15 to 20 minutes

HAVANA-STYLE BLACK BEANS

Serves 6

Ingredients

6 large garlic cloves, chopped

1 tbs. dried oregano

1/4 cup extra virgin olive oil

1 large, western yellow onion, chopped

1 large green bell pepper, cut into 1/2-inch pieces

3 15-to-16 ounce cans black beans, rinsed, drained

3/4 cup Vegetable Broth (use recipe in this section or commercially prepared broth)

1-1/2 tablespoons cider vinegar

Kosher salt and freshly ground pepper, to taste

Directions

1. Heat oil in heavy large saucepan over medium heat

2. Add onion, bell pepper, garlic and oregano and sauté until vegetables begin to soften, about 5 minutes

3. Add 1 cup of beans to pan

4. Using back of fork, mash beans coarsely

5. Add remaining beans, broth and vinegar and simmer until mixture thickens and flavors blend, stirring occasionally, about 15 minutes

6. Season beans to taste with salt and pepper and serve

HERBED AND GRASS-FED FILET MIGNON

Serves 4

Ingredients

4 grass-fed, filet mignon steaks, about 1-1/2 inches thick

4 tbs. extra virgin olive oil

2 cloves garlic, minced

1 tsp. rosemary

1 tsp. thyme

1 tsp. marjoram

1/4 tsp. kosher salt

1/4 tsp. black pepper

Directions

1. Heat olive oil and garlic in a covered microwave safe bowl for 50-60 seconds
2. Remove and allow to cool; add herbs and stir
3. Place filet mignon into a shallow glass dish; pour herb mixture over and turn steaks to coat
4. Cover and let marinate for 1-4 hours in refrigerator
5. Preheat grill for high heat
6. Remove steaks, remove excess oil, and season with salt and pepper
7. Place steaks on grill and cook for 5-6 minutes per side; remove from heat and serve

HUMMUS

Serves 8

Ingredients

2 cups drained, well-cooked or canned chickpeas, liquid reserved

1/2 cup tahini (or, sesame paste), including oil

1/4 cup extra virgin olive oil, plus 1 tbs. extra for drizzling

2 cloves garlic, peeled

Kosher salt and freshly ground black pepper, to taste

1 tablespoon ground cumin or paprika, plus one pinch extra of cumin and paprika for sprinkling

Juice of 1 lemon

Directions

1. Put everything except the extras in a food processor and begin to process

2. Add the chickpea liquid or water as needed to allow the machine to produce a smooth puree

3. Drizzle with the extra olive oil and sprinkle with the extra cumin and paprika

KALE CHIPS

Ingredients

1 head kale, washed and thoroughly dried

2 tbs. extra virgin olive oil

Kosher salt

Directions

1. Preheat the oven to 275 °F.
2. Remove the ribs from the kale and cut into 1 1/2-inch pieces
3. Lay pieces on one or more baking sheets so that there is no doubling on the sheets
4. Toss with the olive oil and salt
5. Bake until crisp, turning the leaves halfway through, about 20 minutes

MEDITERRANEAN WHITE BEAN AND KALE SOUP

Serves 8

Ingredients

32 ounces of low sodium chicken broth, divided

12 ounces of chicken sausage, sliced

1 large western yellow onion, thinly sliced

Kosher salt and ground black pepper to taste

7 cups white beans (cannellini, navy or great northern), cooked and divided

1 bunch kale, stems and tough ribs removed, leaves roughly chopped

Directions

Prepare Sausage:

1. Heat 1/4 cup broth in a large pot over medium heat
2. Add sausage slices and cook, stirring occasionally, until liquid has evaporated and sausage is just browned (approximately 10 minutes)
3. Add onions, salt and pepper and cook, stirring often, until softened, about 10 minutes more
4. If onions begin to stick, add a splash of broth

Purée 3 Cups of Beans (Simultaneously):

1. Put 3 cups beans and 2 cups broth into a blender
2. Purée until smooth then set aside

Complete Soup (Once puree is ready):

1. Add remaining broth to sausage in large pot and bring to a boil, scraping up any browned bits

2. Add kale, reduce heat, cover and simmer, stirring occasionally, until wilted and softened, about 5 minutes

3. Uncover, add remaining 4 cups beans, bean puree, salt and pepper and simmer until hot throughout, about 5 minutes more.

PAN-ROASTED VEGETABLES

Serves 4

Ingredients

1 medium zucchini

1 medium summer squash

1 medium red bell pepper

1 medium yellow bell pepper

1 pound fresh asparagus

1 chopped western yellow onion

3 tablespoons extra virgin olive oil

Kosher salt, to taste

1/2 tsp. black pepper

Directions

1. Preheat the oven to 450 °F.
2. Cut zucchini, squash, pepper, asparagus into bite-sized pieces
3. Place the zucchini, squash, bell peppers, asparagus, and onion in a large roasting pan
4. Toss with the oil, salt, and black pepper
5. Spread vegetables onto roasting pan in a single layer
6. Roast for 30 minutes, stirring occasionally, until the vegetables are lightly browned and tender

PAN-SEARED TUNA WITH AVOCADO SLICES AND CILANTRO SAUCE

Serves 1

Ingredients

2 big handfuls fresh cilantro (or, coriander) leaves, finely chopped

1/2 jalapeno, sliced

1 tsp. fresh ginger, grated

1 garlic clove, grated

2 limes, juiced

2 tbs. soy sauce

Sugar, to taste

Kosher salt and freshly ground black pepper, to taste

4 tbs. extra virgin olive oil, divided

1 (6-ounce) block of sushi-quality tuna

1 ripe avocado, halved, peeled, pitted, and sliced

Directions

1. In a mixing bowl, combine the cilantro, jalapeno, ginger, garlic, lime juice, soy sauce, sugar, salt, pepper, and 2 tbs. of olive oil

2. Stir the ingredients together until well blended

3. Place a skillet over medium-high heat and coat with the remaining 2 tbs. of olive oil

4. Season the tuna generously with salt and pepper

5. Lay the tuna in the hot oil and sear for 1 minute on each side to form a slight crust

6. Pour 1/2 of the cilantro mixture into the pan to coat the tuna
7. Serve the seared tuna with the sliced avocado
8. Drizzle the remaining cilantro sauce over the whole plate

VEGETABLE BROTH

Ingredients

1 pound celery, leaves and insides removed

1-1/2 pounds sweet onions

1 pound carrots, cut into 1 inch pieces

1 pound tomatoes, cored

1 pound green bell pepper, cut into 1-inch pieces

2 tbs. extra virgin olive oil

3 cloves garlic

3 whole cloves leaves

1 bay leaf

6 whole black peppercorns

1 bunch fresh parsley, chopped

1 gallon water

Directions

1. Preheat oven to 450 °F
2. Toss onions, carrots, tomatoes and bell peppers with olive oil
3. Place vegetables in a roasting pan and place them in the oven
4. Stir the vegetable every 15 minutes
5. Cook for over an hour until all of the vegetables have browned and you see signs of the onions caramelizing
6. Put the browned vegetables, celery, garlic, cloves, bay leaf, pepper corns, parsley and water into a large stock pot
7. Bring to a full boil; then simmer

8. Cook uncovered until liquid is reduced by half
9. Pour the broth through a colander, catching the broth in a large bowl or pot

Made in the USA
Lexington, KY
27 December 2014